Atkins Diet Book for Beginners 2024: The ultimate guide to burning belly fat and losing weight. 101 Low-Carb recipes that can help you burn calories.

I0703597

Sébastien Quenneville

Copyright

Copyright © 2024 by Sébastien Quenneville

Disclaimer:

The material offered in this book is for educational and informative purposes only and is not meant as medical advice. The author, Sébastien Quenneville, is not a healthcare practitioner, and the material of this book should not be used as a replacement for professional medical advice, diagnosis, or treatment. Always seek the opinion of your physician or other competent healthcare expert with any queries you may have about a medical condition or food regimen.

The author and publisher of this book make no claims or guarantees with regard to the correctness, application, suitability, or completeness of the contents of this book. The material presented is based on the author's own experiences and research and is subject to change without notice.

The author and publisher disclaim all responsibility, loss, or risk suffered as a result, directly or indirectly, of the use and application of any of the contents of this book. The reader is completely responsible for their own health and wellness, and any dietary or lifestyle modifications should be done in collaboration with a certified healthcare expert.

About the Author

Sébastien Quenneville, originating from France, is a passionate advocate for health and wellbeing, with a deep interest in nutrition and exercise. As a devoted researcher and practitioner, Sébastien has spent years investigating different nutritional methods and lifestyle techniques to promote health and vitality.

Drawing on his own personal experiences and significant study, Sébastien has formed a profound knowledge of the relevance of nutrition in attaining maximum health and wellness. His path towards a healthy living has encouraged him to share his expertise and experiences with others, with the objective of enabling others to take charge of their health and alter their lives.

Sébastien's approach to health and wellness is anchored on a commitment to evidence-based treatments and a comprehensive understanding of wellbeing. He believes in the power of full, nutrient-dense foods to feed the body and promote general health, and he is enthusiastic about helping people find the transformational potential of a healthy diet and lifestyle.

Through his work, Sébastien strives to simplify difficult dietary ideas and give practical, actionable advice that anybody can adopt into their everyday life. His simple, straightforward approach and focus on real-world applications make his work accessible to readers of various backgrounds and levels of experience.

In addition to his writing, Sébastien is also an active chef and recipe creator, always experimenting with new tastes and ingredients to produce tasty, nutritious meals that encourage health and wellbeing. He thinks that eating should be both healthful and pleasant, and he is devoted to sharing his culinary inventions with others.

Sébastien's purpose is to inspire and motivate folks to take care of their health and live their best lives possible. Whether via his writing, cuisine, or personal encounters, he is determined to create a good influence on the lives of people and help them reach their health and wellness objectives.

Table of Contents

Chapter 1: Introduction to the Atkins Diet

This is the Atkins Diet Book for Beginners 2024. Welcome to the book! In the event that you are interested in beginning your path toward a better way of life, you have arrived at the appropriate location. A low-carb approach to eating that has assisted millions of people in achieving their weight reduction and health objectives, the Atkins Diet is the subject of this book, which will walk you through its fundamental concepts.

When it comes to nutrition, the Atkins Diet is not simply another fad diet; rather, it is a scientifically supported strategy that places an emphasis on restricting the amount of carbohydrates you consume in order to maximize your body's capacity to burn fat for fuel. It doesn't matter whether you want to lose a few pounds, boost your energy levels, or just adopt a better way of eating; the Atkins Diet may assist you in accomplishing all of these objectives.

For those who are just starting out on the Atkins Diet, I have gathered together in this book a variety of dishes that are not only easy to make but also very tasty. All the way from scrumptious breakfasts to delectable dinners, decadent desserts to refreshing smoothies, I've got you covered in every single step of the process. In order to guarantee that there is something for everyone, I have even included alternatives for salads, accompaniments, sides, appetizers, and sides, as well as vegetarian and vegan meals.

But this book is not just a compilation of recipes; it is much more than that. I'll also present you with a complete introduction to the Atkins Diet, including its history, concepts, and stages. In this section, I will guide you through the fundamentals of getting started, present you with helpful hints and strategies for achieving success, and suggest resources for more knowledge and assistance.

So whether you're brand new to the Atkins Diet or seeking fresh inspiration to keep you inspired on your path, the Atkins Diet Book for Beginners 2024 is your go-to reference for tasty, fulfilling, and healthful eating. Let's go on this trip together and experience the transformational power of the Atkins Diet!

Brief History of Atkins Diet

The Atkins Diet, designed by Dr. Robert Atkins, exploded onto the scene in the early 1970s and rapidly became one of the most popular and controversial diets of its time. Dr. Atkins, a cardiologist, introduced the world to a novel concept: a low-carbohydrate, high-fat diet as a strategy for weight reduction and enhanced health.

The Atkins Diet questioned traditional understanding about nutrition by calling for a severe decrease in carbohydrate intake while allowing for larger consumption of fats and proteins. Dr. Atkins maintained that by reducing carbs, the body will enter a state of ketosis, when it burns fat for fuel instead of carbohydrates, resulting in fast weight reduction.

Despite receiving opposition from many in the medical and nutritional industries, the Atkins Diet garnered a tremendous following, with millions of individuals claiming considerable weight reduction and improvements in numerous health indices.

Over the years, the Atkins Diet has developed and undergone adjustments, with Dr. Atkins himself issuing revised editions of his original book to reflect new research and ideas. The diet has also generated innumerable spin-offs and modifications, each presenting its unique perspective on low-carb eating.

While the Atkins Diet has encountered criticism for its concentration on saturated fats and possible long-term health hazards, multiple studies have verified its efficacy for weight reduction and addressing specific health issues, such as metabolic syndrome and type 2 diabetes.

Today, the Atkins Diet continues to be a popular option for those looking to reduce weight and improve their health via a low-carb lifestyle. With its focus on genuine, whole foods and flexibility in food choices, the Atkins Diet remains a viable option for anyone hoping to achieve lasting benefits in their quest for greater health and well-being.

Explanation of the principles and phases

The Atkins Diet is built around a set of concepts and stages meant to maximize weight reduction and promote overall health. These concepts and stages constitute the cornerstone of the Atkins method to low-carbohydrate eating, giving a disciplined framework for attaining success on the diet. Here's an explanation of the essential concepts and phases:

1. **Carbohydrate Restriction:**At the basis of the Atkins Diet is the notion of decreasing carbohydrate consumption. Carbohydrates are the body's major source of energy, but when ingested in excess, they may contribute to weight gain and metabolic abnormalities. By reducing carbs, especially those from refined sugars and grains, the body is forced to turn to using fat for fuel, a condition known as ketosis.

2. **stages of the Diet:** The Atkins Diet is split into four stages, each with its own particular principles and objectives:

a. **Induction Phase:**This first phase is the most restricted and normally lasts for two weeks. During this phase, carbohydrate consumption is restricted to 20-25 grams per day, mostly from non-starchy vegetables. The idea is to begin ketosis and stimulate weight reduction.

b. Balancing Phase: In this phase, carbohydrate intake is progressively raised to identify the individual's "Critical Carbohydrate Level for Losing" (CCLL), the greatest quantity of carbs they can ingest while still losing weight. This phase allows for a greater range of meals, including nuts, seeds, and some fruits and vegetables.

c. Pre-Maintenance Phase: Once achieving their weight reduction targets, participants enter the pre-maintenance phase, when carbohydrate consumption is further raised to discover the "Critical Carbohydrate Level for Maintenance" (CCLM). This phase helps sustain weight reduction and prepare for long-term maintenance.

d. Maintenance Phase: The last phase of the Atkins Diet focuses on sustaining weight reduction and supporting general health. Carbohydrate consumption is regulated depending on individual tolerance and metabolic demands, with a focus on complete, nutrient-dense meals.

3. Focus on Protein and Fat: While carbohydrate intake is limited, the Atkins Diet promotes ingestion of protein and healthy fats to offer satiety, maintain muscle maintenance, and power the body. Lean meats, poultry, fish, eggs, nuts, seeds, and oils are cornerstones of the diet, but processed and trans fats are limited.

4. Emphasis on genuine, Whole meals: Unlike many fad diets that depend on packaged and processed meals, the Atkins Diet advocates the intake of genuine, whole foods. This contains lots of non-starchy veggies, coupled with high-quality proteins and fats, to guarantee enough nourishment and promote general health.

Tips for beginners starting the Atkins Diet

Starting any new diet can be both thrilling and hard, particularly if you're new to the Atkins Diet. Here are some crucial guidelines to assist newbies navigate their path and find success on the Atkins Diet:

1. **Educate Yourself:** Take the time to properly learn the fundamentals of the Atkins Diet, including its phases, allowable foods, and suggested parameters. Read books, articles, and trusted websites to educate yourself with the essentials before beginning.

2. **Plan Ahead:** Planning is crucial to success on the Atkins Diet. Before you begin, take some time to plan your meals for the week, including breakfast, lunch, supper, and snacks. Stock your kitchen with lots of low-carb staples, such as lean meats, non-starchy veggies, and healthy fats, to ensure you have plenty of alternatives on hand.

3. **Start Slowly:** If you're new to low-carb eating, try easing into the Atkins Diet gradually, particularly during the induction period. Begin by lowering your carbohydrate consumption gradually over a few days to decrease the possibility of suffering carb withdrawal symptoms.

4. Stay Hydrated: Drinking enough of water is vital on the Atkins Diet, particularly during the induction period when your body is shifting into ketosis. Aim to drink at least eight glasses of water every day to keep hydrated and assist your body's natural detoxifying processes.

5. Monitor Your Progress: Keep note of your food consumption, weight, and measurements periodically to monitor your progress and remain motivated. Consider maintaining a food diary or utilizing a mobile app to log your meals and macros, making it easy to detect any trends or areas for improvement.

6. Focus on Whole Foods: Emphasize genuine, whole foods on the Atkins Diet, such as lean meats, poultry, fish, eggs, nuts, seeds, and non-starchy vegetables. Minimize processed and packaged foods, which may include hidden carbohydrates and bad fats that might derail your efforts.

7. Listen to Your Body: Pay attention to how your body reacts to various meals and change your diet appropriately. Everyone's tolerance for carbs differs, so it's vital to listen to your body's indications and make modifications as required.

8. Seek Support: Joining a group or finding a support system may be immensely useful while beginning the Atkins Diet. Whether it's via online forums, social media groups, or local gatherings, interacting with others who are on a similar path may give support, motivation, and useful insights.

9. **Be Patient and Persistent:** Rome wasn't built in a day, and neither is permanent weight reduction or better health. Be gentle with yourself and trust the process. Remember that improvement takes time, and tiny, persistent adjustments are important to long-term success on the Atkins Diet.

10. **contact with a Healthcare expert:** Before beginning any new diet or lifestyle plan, particularly if you have underlying health ailments or concerns, it's crucial to contact a healthcare expert or registered dietitian. They can give individualized direction and assistance to help you navigate the Atkins Diet safely and efficiently.

Chapter 2: Breakfast Recipes

1. Fennel, Carrot and Turkey Hash Recipe

2. Scrambled Eggs with Bacon, Green Bell Peppers and Tomato Recipe

3. Leek Quiche Recipe

4. Breakfast Berry Parfait Recipe

5. Keto Turkey Breakfast Meatloaf Recipe

6. Eggs with Avocado, Salsa and Turkey Bacon Recipe

7. Keto Scotch Eggs Recipe

8. Eggs Scrambled with Asparagus, Bacon and Swiss Cheese Recipe

9. Eggs Scrambled with Cheddar, Swiss Chard and Canadian Bacon Recipe

10. Cinnamon crumb Coffee Cake Recipe

11. Mushroom Scramble Recipe

12. Keto Mini Chocolate Chip Muffins Recipe

13. Keto Crustless Spinach Quiche Recipe

14. Vegetarian

15. Poached Eggs over Tomato, Avocado and Muenster Recipe

Fennel, Carrot and Turkey Hash Recipe
Prep Time: 10 Minutes
Style: American
Cook Time: 20 Minutes
Difficulty: Difficult

18.1g
Protein

5.2g
Fat

1.5g
Fiber

141.6cal
Calories

INGREDIENTS
   2 tablespoons Canola Vegetable Oil

6 ounces Fennel Bulk 1/2 cup chopped Carrots

3 teaspoons Orange Zest

1/4 cup Freshly Squeezed Orange Juice

1/4 teaspoon Fennel Seed

1 tablespoon Tamari Soybean Sauce

1/2 cup chopped Scallions or Spring Onions12 ounces Turkey Breast Meat (Fryer-Roasters, Cooked, Roasted)

DIRECTIONS

1. Dice the fennel and carrot. In a large pan over medium heat, heat oil; add the fennel and carrot and sauté for approximately 3 minutes. Zest and juice the orange.

2. Add orange zest and juice. Simmer until liquid is nearly absorbed, approximately 4 minutes.

3. Stir in fennel seeds, tamari, onions and chopped turkey. Cook for another 6 minutes until the turkey is cooked through. Top each item with a poached egg if preferred, add 1.3g NC to the total per serving.

Scrambled Eggs with Bacon, Green Bell Peppers and Tomato Recipe

Prep Time: 10 Minutes

Style: American

Cook Time: 10 Minutes

Difficulty: Moderate

24.4g

Protein

22g

Fat

3.5g

Fiber

340.4cal

Calories

INGREDIENTS

- 1 large whole (3" diameter) Red Tomato
- 2 medium slice (yield after cooking) Bacon
- 1/2 cup chopped Green Sweet Pepper
- 2 large Eggs (Whole)
- 1/8 cup shredded Cheddar Cheese

DIRECTIONS

1. Slice tomato into 2-3 thick slices and arrange on a platter. Season with salt and freshly ground black pepper; leave aside.
2. Cook bacon until crispy. Remove excess oil with a paper towel and put over the tomato slices.
3. Sauté chopped green bell pepper for 2-3 minutes in the same skillet as the bacon (drain off excess grease beforehand). Beat the eggs slightly and add them to the green bell peppers. Cook until the eggs are firm.

4. Layer the bacon over the tomatoes, then the eggs. Sprinkle 2 Tbsp cheese on top; broil for one minute or microwave for 30 seconds to melt the cheese.

Leek Quiche Recipe

Prep Time: 15 Minutes

Style: Other

Cook Time: 45 Minutes

Difficulty: Difficult

22.2g

Protein

35.5g

Fat

3.9g

Fiber

490.2cal

Calories

INGREDIENTS

1 tablespoon Unsalted Butter Stick

1 1/2 pounds Leeks

1/2 cup Heavy Cream

3 large Eggs (Whole)

1/2 teaspoon Salt

1/4 teaspoon Black Pepper

1 cup shredded Gruyere Cheese

DIRECTIONS

1. Use 1 Atkins Pie Crust recipe. Follow directions to prebake the pie crust. Prebake the shell and pour filling (directions follow) into the heated shell.

2. Keep the oven on at 350°F. In a medium pan over medium heat, melt butter. Add diced leeks and sauté, stirring periodically, 5 to 6 minutes, until softened. Remove from heat and whisk in cream. Let stand for 5 minutes.

3. Meanwhile, in a larger bowl, mix eggs with salt and pepper. Stir egg mixture into the leeks and cream. Sprinkle ¾ cup of cheese on the bottom of the pie shell.

4. Pour egg mixture into prebaked pie crust; sprinkle remaining cheese on top. Bake for 45 minutes, or until barely set in center and golden on top. If necessary, turn on broiler; broil 6 from element 2 minutes, just until top is browned.

Breakfast Berry Parfait Recipe

Prep Time: 15 Minutes

Style: American

Cook Time: 0 Minutes

Difficulty: Moderate

10.3g

Protein

25.1g
Fat

7.8g
Fiber

337.1cal
Calories

INGREDIENTS

- 2 cups Raspberries
- 1 1/2 cup, wholes Strawberries
- 2 1/2 tablespoons Sucralose Based Sweetener (Sugar Substitute)
- 1 cup Heavy Cream
- 1 tablespoon Vanilla Extract
- 6 ounces Greek Yogurt - Plain (Container)
- 1 bar Atkins Strawberry Shortcake Bar

DIRECTIONS

1. In a blender, purée 1 1/2 cups of the strawberries and 1 1/2 cups of the raspberries with 1 1/2 teaspoons sugar replacement.
2. In a large mixing bowl, using an electric mixer on medium speed, add heavy cream, the remaining 1 tablespoon sugar substitute and the vanilla, whipping to soft peaks. Add yogurt (1 1/2 single serving containers) and whip to firm peaks.

3. In four parfait glasses, alternating layers of the berry mixture, cream filling and crumbled Atkins Strawberry Shortcake Bar, creating at least two layers of each.

4. Top each with part of the remaining 1/2 cup raspberries and serve.

Keto Turkey Breakfast Meatloaf Recipe

Prep Time: 15 Minutes

Style: American

Cook Time: 55 Minutes

Difficulty: Difficult

38.8g

Protein

17.1g

Fat

2.4g

Fiber

340.4cal

Calories

INGREDIENTS

1 10 oz package Frozen Chopped Spinach

4 stalk, medium (7-1/2" - 8" long) Celery

1 medium (approx 2-3/4" long, 2-1/2" diameter) Sweet Red Peppers

24 ounce raw (yield after cooking) Turkey Breakfast Sausage

1 1/2 pounds Ground Turkey

6 large Eggs (Whole)

1 small Onion

1/2 tsp, ground Thyme (Dried)

1 medium (approx 2-3/4" long, 2-1/2" diameter) Green Sweet Pepper

1/8 teaspoon Nutmeg (Ground)

1/8 tablespoon Red or Cayenne Pepper

DIRECTIONS

1. Preheat the oven to 350°F.
2. Thaw the spinach and finely cut. Dice the celery, bell peppers and white onion.
3. Combine the ground turkey sausage and turkey, spinach, celery, bell peppers and onion until completely combined.
4. Add the eggs, thyme, cayenne, nutmeg, 1/2 teaspoon of garlic powder (if wanted) and season with salt and freshly crushed black pepper. Distribute equally and arrange in two standard quick bread pans (4x9 inches).
5. Bake until cooked through and browned on top; approximately 55-65 minutes. Serve immediately or freeze in individual servings for up to 2 months.

Eggs with Avocado, Salsa and Turkey Bacon Recipe

Prep Time: 5 Minutes

Style: American

Cook Time: 15 Minutes

Difficulty: Moderate

31.3g
Protein

39g
Fat

6.3g
Fiber

515.6cal
Calories

INGREDIENTS

- 2 oz, cookeds Turkey Bacon
- 1/2 fruit without skin and seed California Avocados
- 1 ounce Salsa
- 2 large Eggs (Whole)

DIRECTIONS

1. Use the Atkins formula to create Salsa Cruda or use 2 teaspoons of no-sugar-added salsa of your choosing.
2. Cook turkey bacon slices in a non-stick pan over medium-high heat until crispy.
3. Slice avocado.
4. Fry eggs (scramble or poach if wanted instead).

5. Serve the eggs over sliced avocado topped with salsa and the turkey bacon on the side.

Keto Scotch Eggs Recipe

Prep Time: 20 Minutes

Style: Other

Cook Time: 20 Minutes

Difficulty: Difficult

33.5g
Protein

19.8g
Fat

5g
Fiber

361.5cal
Calories

INGREDIENTS

8 large Boiled Eggs

1 large Egg (Whole)

1 teaspoon Tap Water

2 /4 cups Organic High Fiber Coconut Flour

12 ounce raw (yield after cooking) Turkey Breakfast Sausage

DIRECTIONS

1. Prepare hard-boiled eggs. Cover 8 eggs in a heavy pan with 1-inch of cold water. Bring to a rolling boil, remove from the heat and allow eggs to simmer for 10 minutes. Immediately pour off hot water and soak eggs in an ice-water bath until cold enough to peel. Peel eggs and dry well with a paper towel.

2. Whisk 1 egg and water in a small bowl. In another shallow dish lay the coconut flour (season with salt and pepper if required). Set both aside.

3. Prepare sausage by shaping into 8 equal balls. Take each ball and flatten into an oblong disk. Wrap each egg inside the sausage disk being careful to cover the whole surface equally. Set each sausage wrapped egg on a platter.

4. Heat approximately 1-inch of oil in a large frying pan over medium-high heat. Roll each egg in the whisked egg, then the coconut flour until covered all over. When the oil is shimmering, put all 8 eggs (if they fit, allowing at least 1/2-inch in between) in the pan. Fry on one side until golden in color then using tongs flip to another side, continue until both sides are golden brown, roughly 8 minutes total.

5. Drain on a paper towel and serve immediately.

Eggs Scrambled with Asparagus, Bacon and Swiss Cheese Recipe

Prep Time: 5 Minutes

Style: American

Cook Time: 10 Minutes

Difficulty: Moderate

20.6g

Protein

19.6g

Fat

0.7g

Fiber

274.2cal

Calories

INGREDIENTS

- 2 medium slice (yield after cooking) Bacon
- 2 spear, medium (5-1/4" to 7" long) Asparagus
- 1 large Egg (Whole)
- 1 ounce Swiss Cheese

DIRECTIONS

1. Cook bacon in a small skillet over medium high heat. Reserve some of the bacon grease in the pan and discard the remainder or store for later use. Chop bacon into tiny pieces and leave aside.

2. Cook asparagus in a pan with leftover bacon fat until tender, approximately 3 minutes. Remove and cut into bite-size pieces.

3. Add eggs, bacon, cheese and asparagus back to pan and scramble together until egg is done and cheese is melted, approximately 3 minutes. Or skip the cheese and instead sprinkle over the eggs after they are cooked.

4. Season to taste with salt and freshly ground black pepper.

Eggs Scrambled with Cheddar, Swiss Chard and Canadian Bacon Recipe

Prep Time: 5 Minutes

Style: American

Cook Time: 8 Minutes

Difficulty: Moderate

32.6g
Protein

36.9g
Fat

1.2g
Fiber

482.9cal
Calories

INGREDIENTS

1 tablespoon Extra Virgin Olive Oil

2 cups Swiss Chard

2 large Eggs (Whole)

1/4 cup shredded Cheddar Cheese

2 ounces Canadian-Style Bacon (Cured)

DIRECTIONS

1. Sauté Swiss chard in 1 tsp oil until reduced in volume and soft.

2. Beat eggs slightly and add to the pan with Swiss chard. Using a spatula stir to incorporate and heat until eggs are set.

3. Add shredded Cheddar cheese and Canadian bacon on top or it may be tossed in with the eggs and cooked all together.

Cinnamon Crumb Coffee Cake Recipe

Prep Time: 30 Minutes

Style: American

Cook Time: 40 Minutes

Difficulty: Difficult

6.7g

Protein

34.7g

Fat

3.1g

Fiber

383 cal

Calories

INGREDIENTS

- 3/4 cup 100% Stone Ground Whole Wheat Pastry Flour
- 3/4 cup Whole Grain Soy Flour
- 1/2 cup Whole Wheat Flour
- 1 teaspoon Baking Powder (Straight Phosphate, Double Acting)
- 1 teaspoon Baking Soda
- 1/2 teaspoon Salt
- 2 large Eggs (Whole)
- 1 teaspoon Vanilla Extract
- 1 cup Sour Cream (Cultured)
- 1 1/4 cups Unsalted Butter Stick
- 2 cups Sucralose Based Sweetener (Sugar Substitute)
- 1/2 cup, dry, yield Oatmeal
- 1 1/2 cup, halves Pecan Nuts
- 2 teaspoons Cinnamon

DIRECTIONS

1. Preheat the oven to 350°F. Grease a 9x13 inch baking pan and leave aside.

2. For cake: In a medium bowl, mix together pastry flour, soy flour, whole-wheat flour, baking powder, baking soda and salt. In a large liquid measuring cup mix eggs, vanilla and sour cream until completely incorporated.

3. In a large bowl, using an electric mixer on medium speed, beat 1/2 cup butter and 1 cup sugar substitute until creamy and fluffy, approximately 4 minutes. Alternately add the flour mixture and egg mixture to the butter, starting and finishing with the flour mixture.

4. For topping: In a blender, pulse oats, 1 cup sugar substitute, pecans, 3/4 cup butter and cinnamon until texture approaches a coarse meal.

5. To assemble cake: Spread two-thirds of the batter into the prepared pan. Sprinkle half the topping over the batter and softly swirl with a knife to create pockets of topping inside the batter.

6. Spoon remaining batter over topping, and sprinkle evenly with remaining topping. Bake until a knife inserted in the middle comes out clean, approximately 40 minutes. Cool cake in a pan put on a wire rack. Serve heated or at room temperature. Makes 12 servings.

Mushroom Scramble Recipe

Prep Time: 10 Minutes

Style: American

Cook Time: 6 Minutes

Difficulty: Moderate

11.7g

Protein

14.2g

Fat

0.8g

Fiber

192.9cal

Calories

INGREDIENTS

- 1 cup Mushroom Pieces and Stems
- 1/2 cup chopped Onions
- 3 tablespoons Extra Virgin Olive Oil
- 14 ounces Firm Silken Tofu
- 1 cup Baby Spinach
- 1/4 cup shredded Cheddar Cheese
- 3 tablespoons Parmesan Cheese (Grated)
- 4 large Eggs (Whole)
- 1/8 teaspoon leaf Dried Thyme Leaves
- 8 Cherry Tomatoes

DIRECTIONS

1. In a large nonstick skillet, over medium-high heat, sauté the white onion and mushrooms in the oil until tender (approximately 3 minutes).
2. Add the tofu and spinach and simmer for an additional 3 minutes.

3. Stir in the tomatoes, eggs, Cheddar and Parmesan cheeses and 1/8 tsp thyme and heat until the egg is hard.
4. Serve immediately.

Keto Mini Chocolate Chip Muffins Recipe

Prep Time: 10 Minutes

Style: American

Cook Time: 15 Minutes

Difficulty: Difficult

1.7g

Protein

5.2g

Fat

2.1g

Fiber

64.7cal

Calories

INGREDIENTS

2/3 cup Almond Flour, Blanched

1/2 cup Sucralose Based Sweetener (Sugar Substitute)

1/3 cup Coconut Flour

1 teaspoon Baking Powder (Straight Phosphate, Double Acting)

3/4 teaspoon Xanthan Gum

1/4 teaspoon Salt

1/2 cup Sour Cream (Cultured)

2 tablespoons Unsalted Butter Stick

2 tablespoons Heavy Cream

1 fluid ounce Tap Water

2 teaspoons Vanilla Extract

4 ounces Lily's Sugar Free Chocolate Chips

DIRECTIONS

1. Heat oven to 350°F. Grease 24 mini muffin wells, or line with mini muffin paper liners.

2. In a bowl, add almond flour, sugar replacement, coconut flour, baking powder, xanthan gum, and salt.

3. In another dish, stir sour cream, melted butter, heavy cream, water and vanilla to blend.

4. Add the sour cream mixture to the flour mixture. Stir until completely blended. Fold in chocolate chips.

5. Fill muffin wells equally with a scant 1 tablespoon each muffin. Bake for 20 minutes, or until gently browned on top and the toothpick inserted in the middle comes out clean.

6. Cool muffins in pans for 5 minutes, then flip out onto wire racks to cool fully.

Keto Crustless Spinach Quiche Recipe

Prep Time: 20 Minutes

Style: French

Cook Time: 30 Minutes

Difficulty: Difficult

16.1g

Protein

38.1g

Fat

2.1g

Fiber

427.3cal

Calories

INGREDIENTS

- 2 teaspoons Canola Vegetable Oil
- 1/2 cup chopped Scallions or Spring Onions
- 6 1/2 ounces Frozen Chopped Spinach
- 4 large Eggs (Whole)
- 1 cup Heavy Cream
- 1 cup shredded Muenster Cheese
- 1/4 teaspoon Salt
- 1/4 teaspoon Black Pepper
- 1/8 teaspoon Nutmeg (Ground)

DIRECTIONS

1. Preheat the oven to 350°F (175°C). Lightly oil a 9 inch pie pan.

2. Heat oil in a large skillet over medium-high heat. Add onions and simmer, turning periodically, until onions are tender. Cut frozen spinach into bits, add to pan and continue cooking until spinach is heated through and extra liquid has disappeared.

3. In a large bowl, mix eggs, cream, cheese, salt, pepper and nutmeg. Add spinach mixture and toss to incorporate. Pour into the prepared pie pan.

4. Bake in a preheated oven until eggs have set, approximately 30 minutes. Let cool for 10 minutes before serving.

5. If using fresh spinach, add chopped spinach (or whole baby spinach) to the skillet with the onions two cups at a time with a tablespoon of water, cooking until the spinach begins to wilt before adding another 2 cups, until all spinach is wilted and moisture has evaporated before adding it to the egg mixture.

Vegetarian

Prep Time: 5 Minutes

Style: American

Cook Time: 0 Minutes

Difficulty: Moderate

29.6g

Protein

13.1g

Fat

4g

Fiber

266 cal

Calories

INGREDIENTS

1 1/2 servings Smart Deli Roast Turkey Style

1 slice (1 ounce) Swiss Cheese

3 spear, medium (5-1/4" to 7" long) Asparagus

DIRECTIONS

1. Lay down 2 slices of "turkey" then one piece of Swiss cheese.

2. Place 1 asparagus spear at one end and roll-up. Pin with a toothpick if desired.

3. Repeat with remaining ingredients.

Poached Eggs over Tomato, Avocado and Muenster Recipe

Prep Time: 5 Minutes

Style: American

Cook Time: 5 Minutes

Difficulty: Moderate

21.3g

Protein

31.9g

Fat

6.4g

Fiber

403.1cal

Calories

INGREDIENTS

2 large Eggs (Whole)

1/3 medium whole (2-3/5" diameter) Red Tomatoes

1/2 fruit without skin and seed California Avocados

1 ounce Muenster Cheese

DIRECTIONS

1. Poach eggs: add 2 to 3 inches of water with a bit of salt to a pot. Bring to a boil; then turn down heat and let water simmer until hardly any bubbles remain around the rims. Crack an egg into a cup and delicately slide it into the water. Cook 2 minutes for a runny yolk, 3 minutes for medium firmness and 4 minutes for a hard yolk. Remove with a slotted spoon. Gently pat with a paper towel to remove excess water.

2. Slice tomato and avocado. Place tomato slices on a platter, top with avocado, cheese and lastly the eggs.

3. Sprinkle with paprika (if preferred), and season to taste with salt and freshly ground black pepper.

Chapter 3: Lunch recipes

16. Salmon Stuffed Avocados

17. Spinach & Artichoke-Stuffed Portobello Mushrooms

18. Mozzarella, Basil & Zucchini Frittata

19. Turkey & Cheddar Lettuce Wraps

20. Taco Lettuce Wraps

21. Pickle Sub Sandwiches with Turkey & Cheddar

22. Spinach & Mushroom Quiche

23. Barbecue Chicken Kale Wraps

Salmon Stuffed Avocados

Prep Time: 15

Total Time: 15

Servings: 4

23g
Protein

20g
Fat

11g
Carbs

293 cal

Calories

INGREDIENTS

½ cup nonfat plain Greek yogurt

½ cup diced celery

2 tablespoons chopped fresh parsley

1 tablespoon lime juice

2 teaspoons mayonnaise

1 teaspoon Dijon mustard

⅛ teaspoon salt

⅛ teaspoon ground pepper

2 (5 ounce) cans salmon, drained, flaked, skin and bones removed

2 avocados

Chopped chives for garnish

DIRECTIONS

1. Combine yogurt, celery, parsley, lime juice, mayonnaise, mustard, salt, and pepper in a medium bowl; mix well. Add salmon and combine thoroughly.

2. Halve avocados lengthwise and remove pits. Scoop roughly 1 tablespoon flesh from each avocado half into a small dish. Mash the scooped-out avocado flesh with a fork and add into the salmon mixture.

3. Fill each avocado half with approximately 1/4 cup of the salmon mixture, mounding it on top of the avocado halves. Garnish with chives, if desired.

Spinach & Artichoke-Stuffed Portobello Mushrooms

Prep Time:

30 mins

Total Time:

30 mins

Servings:

4

Yield:

4 mushrooms

8g

Protein

11g

Fat

14g

Carbs

175 cal

Calories

INGREDIENTS

2 tablespoons extra-virgin olive oil

1 teaspoon garlic powder, divided

½ teaspoon ground pepper, divided

⅛ teaspoon salt, divided

4 large portobello mushrooms (about 14 ounces), stems and gills removed (see Tip)

1 (5 ounce) package baby spinach, roughly chopped

1 (14 ounce) can artichoke hearts, rinsed, squeezed dry and chopped

2 ounces reduced-fat cream cheese, softened

¼ cup grated Parmesan cheese, plus more for garnish

DIRECTIONS

1. Preheat the oven to 400 degrees F.

2. Combine oil, garlic powder, 1/4 teaspoon pepper and 1/8 teaspoon salt in a small bowl. Using a silicone brush, cover mushrooms all over with the oil mixture. Place on a large rimmed baking sheet and bake until the mushrooms are mostly cooked, approximately 10 minutes.

3. Meanwhile, mix spinach and 1 tablespoon water in a large skillet over medium heat. Cook, tossing occasionally, until barely wilted, approximately 2 minutes. Drain as much water as possible from the spinach, then transfer to a medium bowl. Add artichokes, cream cheese, Parmesan and the remaining 1/4 teaspoon pepper and 1/8 teaspoon salt. Stir well to mix. Divide the mixture between the mushrooms and bake until heated, 7 to 10 minutes.

Mozzarella, Basil & Zucchini Frittata
Cook Time:
20 mins

Total Time:

20 mins

Servings:

4

18g

Protein

21g

Fat

8g

Carbs

292 cal

Calories

INGREDIENTS

  2 tablespoons extra-virgin olive oil

  1 ½ cups thinly sliced red onion

  1 ½ cups chopped zucchini

  7 large eggs, beaten

  ½ teaspoon salt

  ¼ teaspoon freshly ground pepper

  ⅔ cup pearl-size or baby fresh mozzarella balls (about 4 ounces)

  3 tablespoons chopped soft sun-dried tomatoes

  ¼ cup thinly sliced fresh basil

DIRECTIONS

1. Position rack in top third of oven; preheat broiler.

2. Heat oil in a large broiler-safe nonstick or cast-iron pan over medium-high heat. Add onion and zucchini and cook, stirring constantly, until tender, 3 to 5 minutes.

3. Meanwhile, mix eggs, salt and pepper in a bowl. Pour the eggs over the veggies in the pan. Cook, raising the sides to allow raw egg from the center to run below, until almost set, approximately 2 minutes. Arrange mozzarella and sun-dried tomatoes on top and set the pan on the broiler until the eggs are slightly browned, 1 1/2 to 2 minutes. Let stand for 3 minutes. Top with basil.

4. To remove the frittata from the pan, run a spatula along the edge, then beneath, until you can slide or lift it out onto a cutting board or serving dish. Cut into 4 pieces and serve.

Turkey & Cheddar Lettuce Wraps
Prep Time: 15 mins
Total Time: 15 mins
Servings: 4
Yield: 4 wraps

21g

Protein

22g

Fat

3g

Carbs

324 cal

Calories

INGREDIENTS

¼ cup mayonnaise

3 tablespoons chopped dill pickle

2 teaspoons whole-grain mustard

8 large green-leaf lettuce leaves

12 ounces sliced deli turkey

4 ounces sliced deli sharp Cheddar cheese

8 slices tomato

DIRECTIONS

1. Stir mayonnaise, pickle and mustard together in a small bowl.

2. Overlap 2 lettuce leaves on a clean cutting board. Spread a liberal 1 spoonful of the mayonnaise mixture over the lettuce. Top with 3 ounces turkey, 1 ounce cheese and 2 tomato slices. Roll into a wrap, then cut in half. Repeat with the remaining ingredients.

Taco Lettuce Wraps

Cook Time: 30 mins

Total Time: 30 mins

Servings: 4

23g
Protein

19g
Fat

8g
Carbs

291 cal
Calories

INGREDIENTS

8 small iceberg or romaine lettuce leaves or 4 large, cut in half crosswise

1 tablespoon canola oil

1 pound lean ground beef

¼ teaspoon salt

5 tablespoons prepared salsa

1 tablespoon rice vinegar

1 ½ teaspoons ground cumin

1 cup diced avocado

1 cup julienned jícama (see Tip)

¼ cup finely diced red onion

DIRECTIONS

1. Wash and dry lettuce leaves carefully and take off any tough ribs.

2. Heat oil in a large nonstick skillet over medium-high heat. Add ground beef, season with salt and heat, turning constantly, until cooked through, 4 to 6 minutes.

3. Meanwhile, combine salsa, vinegar and cumin in a small basin.

4. Remove the pan from the heat, add the salsa mixture and toss to incorporate. Serve in the lettuce leaves, topped with avocado, jicama and onion.

Pickle Sub Sandwiches with Turkey & Cheddar
Prep Time: 10 mins
Total Time: 10 mins
Servings: 4
Yield: 4 sandwiches

12g
Protein

12g
Fat

4g
Carbs

186 cal

Calories

INGREDIENTS

8 large kosher dill pickle slices (sandwich stackers)

2 teaspoons mayonnaise

4 ounces deli roast turkey slices

4 (1 ounce) slices Cheddar cheese, halved

8 slices Roma tomato

4 small romaine lettuce leaves

DIRECTIONS

Pat pickle slices dry with paper towels. Spread 1/2 teaspoon mayonnaise on each of 4 pickle slices. Top each with 1 ounce turkey, 2 pieces of Cheddar, 2 tomato slices and 1 lettuce leaf. Top with a simple pickle slice.

Spinach & Mushroom Quiche

Active Time: 25 mins

Total Time: 1 hr 5 mins

Servings: 6

Yield: 1 quiche

17g

Protein

20g

Fat

7g
Carbs

277 cal
Calories

INGREDIENTS

2 tablespoons extra-virgin olive oil

8 ounces sliced fresh mixed wild mushrooms such as cremini, shiitake, button and/or oyster mushrooms

1 ½ cups thinly sliced sweet onion

1 tablespoon thinly sliced garlic

5 ounces fresh baby spinach (about 8 cups), coarsely chopped

6 large eggs

¼ cup whole milk

¼ cup half-and-half

1 tablespoon Dijon mustard

1 tablespoon fresh thyme leaves, plus more for garnish

¼ teaspoon salt

¼ teaspoon ground pepper

1 ½ cups shredded Gruyère cheese

DIRECTIONS

Preheat the oven to 375 degrees F. Coat a 9-inch pie tin with cooking spray; put aside.

Heat oil in a large nonstick skillet over medium-high heat; swirl to coat the pan. Add mushrooms; cook, turning occasionally, until browned and soft, approximately 8 minutes. Add onion and garlic; cook, turning regularly, until softened and tender, approximately 5 minutes. Add spinach; cook, stirring regularly, until wilted, 1 to 2 minutes. Remove from heat.

3. Whisk eggs, milk, half-and-half, mustard, thyme, salt and pepper in a larger bowl. Fold in the mushroom mixture and cheese. Spoon into the prepared pie pan. Bake until firm and golden brown, approximately 30 minutes. Let stand for 10 minutes; slice. Garnish with thyme and serve.

Barbecue Chicken Kale Wraps
Cook Time: 30 mins
Total Time: 30 mins
Servings: 4

24g
Protein

7g
Fat

15g
Carbs

216 cal

Calories

INGREDIENTS

8 small kale leaves or 4 large, cut in half crosswise

1 tablespoon canola oil

1 pound boneless, skinless chicken breast, trimmed and cut into bite-size pieces

¼ teaspoon salt

5 tablespoons prepared barbecue sauce

1 tablespoon rice vinegar

1 ½ teaspoons Cajun seasoning

1 cup thinly sliced red cabbage

1 cup julienned carrots

¼ cup thinly sliced scallion greens

DIRECTIONS

1. Wash and dry kale leaves carefully; take off any stiff ribs or stems.
2. Heat oil in a large nonstick skillet over medium-high heat. Add chicken, season with salt and heat, tossing regularly, until cooked through, 4 to 6 minutes.
3. Meanwhile, combine barbecue sauce, vinegar and Cajun spice in a small basin.
4. Remove the skillet from the heat, add the sauce mixture and toss to incorporate. Serve in the kale leaves, topped with cabbage, carrots and scallion greens.

Chapter 4: Dinner Recipes

24. White Pizza with Broccoli Recipe

 25. Chicken and Cheese Quesadillas Recipe

26. Turkey Tacos Recipe

27. Curried Fish and Red Peppers Over Broccoli Recipe

28. Lettuce-Wrapped Swiss Cheeseburger with Tomato and Hummus Recipe

29. Tofu Sautéed with Green Pepper, Scallions and Tamari Recipe

30. Keto Beef Burger with Feta and Tomato Recipe

31.Keto Baked Tofu with Cajun Rub Recipe

32. Keto Tequila Chicken Recipe

33. Wild Salmon Vera Cruz with Grilled Asparagus and Watercress Recipe

34. Double Mushroom Soup Recipe

35. Roasted Vegetable Soup Recipe

White Pizza with Broccoli Recipe

Prep Time: 10 Minutes

Style: Italian

Cook Time: 10 Minutes

Difficulty: Difficult

30.2g

Protein

21.8g

Fat

5.6g

Fiber

372.8cal

Calories

INGREDIENTS

   1 package Bakers Yeast (Active Dry)

   1 1/2 cups (8 fluid ounces) Water

   2 1/2 cups Whole Grain Soy Flour

   4 ounces Vital Wheat Gluten

   1 1/2 teaspoons Baking Powder (Sodium Aluminum Sulfate, Double Acting)

   1/4 teaspoon Salt

   5 tablespoons Olive Oil

   2 cloves Garlic

   1 pound Broccoli

   3/4 cup Ricotta Cheese (Whole Milk)

1/2 cup shredded Mozzarella Cheese (Whole Milk)

4 tablespoons Parmesan Cheese (Grated)

1 teaspoon Oregano

DIRECTIONS

1. Prepare a 14-inch pizza pan with air holes by spraying gently with oil. Set aside. Combine yeast with 1/2 cup warm water in a small dish. Set alone for a few minutes to get frothy.

2. In a large basin mix to incorporate the soy flour, wheat gluten, baking powder and salt. Add the warm yeast water and 3 tbsp olive oil mixing with your hands. Slowly add additional water a tablespoon at a time until it produces a workable dough. Place into an oiled bowl and cover with plastic wrap. Place in a warm location and let it double in size for 1 hour. Remove plastic wrap, punch down, flatten and reshape into the pizza pan. While the dough is rising, create the topping.

3. Preheat the oven to 450°F.

4. For the topping: Heat 1 tbsp olive oil in a pan over medium heat. Mince the garlic and add it to the pan, fry for 30 seconds then add the chopped broccoli and simmer for another 2 minutes. Remove from heat and add the ricotta cheese, stirring until mixed. Spread mixture over the crust leaving a 1/2-inch border then top with mozzarella and Parmesan cheeses.

5. Sprinkle with oregano and remaining 1 tbsp of oil. Bake for 20-22 minutes until puffed and nicely browned.

Chicken and Cheese Quesadillas Recipe

Prep Time: 5 Minutes

Style: Mexican

Cook Time: 5 Minutes

Difficulty: Moderate

34g

Protein

27.6g

Fat

8.3g

Fiber

418.5cal

Calories

INGREDIENTS

- 1 cup shredded Monterey Jack Cheese
- 8 tortillas Low Carb Tortillas
- 8 ounces boneless, cooked Chicken Breast
- 2 ounces Roasted Bell Peppers
- 3 medium (4-1/8" long) Scallions or Spring Onions
- 4 sprigs Cilantro
- 3 tablespoons Unsalted Butter Stick

DIRECTIONS

1. Divide and put half of the cheese on 4 tortillas, leaving a 1/2-inch border around the edge. Dice the chicken, roasted peppers and scallions. Evenly divide into four halves then lay over the cheese. Sprinkle it with cilantro and remaining cheese. Cover each with a tortilla.

2. Heat two big nonstick skillets over medium-high heat for 2 minutes. Add one slice of butter to each pan, and heat until melted. Place one quesadilla in each pan, and cook for 2 to 3 minutes each side, rotating gently with a broad spatula. Repeat with remaining butter and quesadillas.

3. Cut each tortilla into eight wedges. If desired, sprinkle with sour cream, salsa, tiny bell pepper and jalapeño (but note this will add extra carbohydrates).

Turkey Tacos Recipe

Prep Time: 10 Minutes

Style: American

Cook Time: 10 Minutes

Difficulty: Difficult

39.5g
Protein

17.7g
Fat

4.8g

Fiber

356.7cal
Calories

INGREDIENTS

2 tablespoons Light Olive Oil

16 oz, boneless, cooked, skinlesses Turkey Cutlet

1 tablespoon Original Taco Seasoning Mix

1/3 cup Sour Cream (Cultured)

1/4 cup chopped Red Onions

1 ounce Cilantro (Coriander)

4 tortillas Low Carb Tortillas

1/2 medium (approx 2-3/4" long, 2-1/2" diameter) Green Sweet Pepper

2 ounces Salsa

DIRECTIONS

1. Heat 1 tablespoon (3 tablespoons) oil in a large pan over medium-high heat. Sprinkle turkey cutlets with taco seasoning and sauté until barely cooked through, approximately 2 minutes each side. Transfer turkey to a chopping board and cut into strips.

2. Add sour cream, onion and cilantro to the skillet. Cook until onions are slightly softened and mixture is cooked through, approximately 3 minutes.

3. Return turkey strips and any collected juices to the skillet, stir to coat and remove from heat.

4. To create each taco, heat 1 teaspoon of oil in a medium pan over high heat until extremely hot. Add tortilla and cook for 1 minute each side until light golden brown. Remove and drain excess oil on paper towels. Place 1/4 of the filling on half of the tortilla, fold and top with 1/4 of the pepper strips and 1 tablespoon salsa. Repeat the entire process with remaining tortillas.

Curried Fish and Red Peppers Over Broccoli Recipe

Prep Time: 10 Minutes

Style: Asian

Cook Time: 15 Minutes

Difficulty: Difficult

43.3g
Protein

17.5g
Fat

0.9g
Fiber

354.3cal
Calories

INGREDIENTS

32 ounces Tilapia

6 cup florets Broccoli Flower Clusters

1 1/2 cups Coconut Cream, canned

1/2 tablespoon Roasted Red Chili Paste

2 teaspoons Ginger

1 1/2 tablespoons Fish Sauce

3 teaspoons Sucralose Based Sweetener (Sugar Substitute)

3 cups sliced Red Sweet Pepper

1/2 fluid ounce Fresh Lime Juice

DIRECTIONS

1. Lightly season fish with salt and freshly ground black pepper. Set aside.

2. Prepare a medium pot to boil water equipped with a steamer basket. Once the water boils, steam the broccoli until it is crisp-tender; around 5-10 minutes. While broccoli is steaming, make the fish and sauce.

3. In a large sauté pan over medium-high heat add the coconut milk, chili paste, chopped ginger, lime juice, fish sauce, granular sugar replacement and bell peppers. Mix to mix sauce ingredients, continue to heat till it boils then add the fish. Cook the fish using the sauce to baste every 2-3 minutes until the flesh is opaque and flakes easily. Remove fish to a platter and continue to reduce sauce over the heat until it thickens slightly. Return fish to pan to rewarm 2-3 minutes, add the lime juice and serve immediately over the broccoli.

Lettuce-Wrapped Swiss Cheeseburger with Tomato and Hummus Recipe

Prep Time: 5 Minutes

Style: American

Cook Time: 10 Minutes

Difficulty: Moderate

42.2g

Protein

47.3g

Fat

2.3g

Fiber

647.7cal

Calories

INGREDIENTS

- 5 ounces Ground Beef (80% Lean / 20% Fat)
- 2 slice (1 ounce) Swiss Cheese
- 1 small whole (2-2/5" diameter) Red Tomato
- 2 tablespoons Organic Hummus Classic
- 3 leaves Butterhead Lettuce (Includes Boston and Bibb Types)

DIRECTIONS

1. Season hamburger patty with salt and freshly ground black pepper. Grill burger to desired doneness, approximately 5 minutes each side.
2. Top with Swiss cheese the final few minutes of cooking to melt.
3. Top with tomato and hummus.
4. Wrap with lettuce leaves.

Tofu Sautéed with Green Pepper, Scallions and Tamari Recipe

Prep Time: 5 Minutes

Style: Asian

Cook Time: 10 Minutes

Phase: Phase 2

Difficulty: Moderate

11.7g

Protein

16.8g

Fat

3.3g

Fiber

243 cal

Calories

INGREDIENTS

1 tablespoon Extra Virgin Olive Oil

4 ounces Firm Silken Tofu

3/4 cup chopped Green Sweet Pepper

1/2 cup chopped Scallions or Spring Onions

1 tablespoon Tamari Soybean Sauce

DIRECTIONS

1. Heat oil in a nonstick skillet over medium-high heat. Add tofu and sauté for 5 minutes, flipping several times until golden brown.
2. Add green peppers and scallions and sauté 3-4 minutes until veggies are cooked.
3. Season with tamari during the final minute of cooking. Serve immediately.

Keto Beef Burger with Feta and Tomato Recipe

Prep Time: 10 Minutes

Style: American

Cook Time: 12 Minutes

Phase: Phase 1

Difficulty: Moderate

21.2g

Protein

24.7g

Fat

0.5g

Fiber

318.7cal

Calories

INGREDIENTS

- 1 pound Ground Beef (80% Lean / 20% Fat)
- 1 large Scallions or Spring Onion
- 1/2 cup Baby Spinach
- 1/4 cup, chopped or sliced Red Tomatoes
- 1/4 cup, crumbled Feta Cheese
- 1/2 teaspoon Dill weed, dried
- 1/2 teaspoon Salt
- 1/2 teaspoon Black Pepper

DIRECTIONS

1. Combine ground beef, scallion, spinach, tomato, feta, 1.5 tsp fresh dill (or 1/2 tsp dried), salt and pepper. Form into 4 patties.
2. Grill or pan-fry over medium-high heat for 6 minutes each side for medium doneness.

Keto Baked Tofu with Cajun Rub Recipe

Prep Time: 5 Minutes

Style: American

Cook Time: 30 Minutes

Phase: Phase 1

Difficulty: Moderate

12.4g

Protein

9.6g

Fat

1.7g

Fiber

160 cal

Calories

INGREDIENTS

- 1 serving Keto Cajun Rub
- 6 ounces Firm Silken Tofu
- 1 teaspoon Extra Virgin Olive Oil

DIRECTIONS

1. Use the Atkins recipe to make Cajun Rub, you will need 1 tablespoon.
2. Drain and pat tofu dry with a paper towel. Cut into 1/4 inch strips. Rub spice and oil over tofu and marinate for 30 minutes if preferred. Or put spice onto tofu and cook immediately.
3. Preheat oven to 375°

4. Bake on an oiled flat pan for 15 minutes, flip over and bake an extra 15 minutes until golden brown and somewhat crispy.

Keto Tequila Chicken Recipe

Prep Time: 10 Minutes

Style: Mexican

Cook Time: 15 Minutes

Phase: Phase 1

Difficulty: Difficult

36.2g

Protein

48.6g

Fat

0.4g

Fiber

613.3cal

Calories

INGREDIENTS

1/2 cup Canola Oil

1/4 cup Cilantro (Coriander)

1 1/2 fluid ounce (no ice) Tequila

1 1/2 tablespoons Cumin

3 teaspoons Garlic

1 teaspoon Salt

1/2 teaspoon Black Pepper

1/8 teaspoon Red or Cayenne Pepper

32 ounce raw (yield after cooking, bone removed) Chicken Breast

1/4 cup Unsalted Butter Stick

DIRECTIONS

1. Heat oven 400°F.

2. In a large bowl, add oil, cilantro, tequila, cumin, garlic, salt, pepper and cayenne. Add chicken and toss to coat.

3. Transfer chicken to a baking sheet. Bake for 12 to 14 minutes, or until the biggest piece is cooked through.

4. Remove from the oven and top each breast with a tiny dollop of butter and let it melt.

Wild Salmon Vera Cruz with Grilled Asparagus and Watercress Recipe

Prep Time: 20 Minutes

Style: Mexican

Cook Time: 10 Minutes

Phase: Phase 2

Difficulty: Difficult

27.1g

Protein

59.2g

Fat

7.9g

Fiber

732.8cal

Calories

INGREDIENTS

12 spear, medium (5-1/4" to 7" long) Asparagus

7 tablespoons Extra Virgin Olive Oil

1 teaspoon Salt

1 teaspoon Black Pepper

1 pound Wild Atlantic Salmon

1/2 cup chopped Sweet Red Peppers

10 cloves Garlic

1/2 cup chopped Onions

3 medium whole (2-3/5" diameter) Tomatoes

8 fluid ounces Sauvignon Blanc Wine

20 10 smalls Green Olives

2 tablespoons Butter

2 cups chopped Watercress

DIRECTIONS

The salmon is pan roasted, providing for quick clean-up. While the taste of wild salmon is excellent, a less costly option is farm-raised salmon. The trade winds of Spain went straight to Vera Cruz, where the local people absorbed European items like olives, capers and other dishes into their diet, giving it a European taste.

1. Preheat the grill or broiler.
2. Toss the asparagus stalks with 3 tablespoons of virgin olive oil and salt & pepper. Grill until barely tender, approximately 3-4 minutes, rolling regularly. Set aside and keep heated.
3. Meanwhile, rinse and spin dry the watercress. Set aside.
4. Heat 3 tablespoons of the olive oil in a large sauté pan or skillet over medium-high heat.
5. Sprinkle the fish with salt and pepper. Place it in the pan flesh side down, and sear until golden, approximately 2–3 minutes. Flip the salmon over.
6. Add the bell peppers, thinly sliced garlic, onions, diced tomatoes and wine to the pan; bring to a simmer. Cook, uncovered, until the salmon is medium rare, approximately 4-5 minutes.
7. Add the olives and butter, stirring the butter continually until it is integrated; check the spices and add more salt and pepper to taste.
8. Toss the watercress with 1 tablespoon extra-virgin olive oil and salt.
9. To serve, arrange 3 stalks of asparagus on each dish. Top with a slice of salmon and one-quarter of the sauce, spreading it out evenly. Add one-quarter of the watercress to each dish.

Double Mushroom Soup Recipe

Prep Time: 35 Minutes

Style: American

Cook Time: 45 Minutes

Difficulty: Difficult

12.3g

Protein

16g

Fat

1.2g

Fiber

217.7cal

Calories

INGREDIENTS

5 pieces Dried Porcini Mushrooms

4 cans (10.75 ounces), prepared to directions Chicken Broth, Bouillon or Consomme

3 tablespoons Unsalted Butter Stick

1 small Onion

12 ounces Mushroom Pieces and Stems

3 teaspoons Garlic

3 tablespoons Atkins Flour mix

1 teaspoon Thyme

1/4 teaspoon Nutmeg (Ground)

1/2 cup Heavy Cream

DIRECTIONS

Use the Atkins recipe to produce Atkins Flour Mix for this dish.

1. In a dish, cover porcinis with 14 1/2 ounces chicken broth; let stand for 30 minutes. Strain the soaking liquid; put aside. Roughly slice porcinis; put aside.

2. Melt butter in a pot over medium heat. Add chopped onion and sliced button mushrooms and sauté for 10 minutes. Add minced garlic and sauté for another 30 seconds. Add 3 tablespoons Atkins Flour Mix; mix and simmer for 2 minutes. Gradually mix in remaining 29 ounces of chicken broth, saved porcini liquid, thyme and nutmeg. Increase heat to high and bring to a boil; lower heat to medium-low and simmer for 5 minutes. Add chopped porcinis to soup; simmer 10 more minutes until softened.

3. Blend half the soup in a blender or food processor until smooth and return to the pot. Add cream and boil soup for 3 minutes. Season with salt and pepper to taste.

Roasted Vegetable Soup Recipe

Prep Time: 20 Minutes

Style: Other

Cook Time: 75 Minutes

Difficulty: Difficult

4.9g

Protein

17.3g

Fat

5.6g

Fiber

212.3cal

Calories

INGREDIENTS

- 4 plum tomatoes Red Tomatoes
- 2 eggplant, unpeeled (approx 1-1/4 lb) Eggplant
- 4 cloves Garlic
- 3 tablespoons Light Olive Oil
- 1 1/4 teaspoons Marjoram (Dried)
- 2 14.5 ounces cans Chicken Broth, Bouillon or Consomme
- 1 cup Heavy Cream
- 3/4 teaspoon Salt
- 1/2 teaspoon Black Pepper
- 6 large Scallions or Spring Onions

DIRECTIONS

1. Heat oven to 400°F.
2. Place tomatoes, eggplants, green onions and garlic in a shallow roasting pan. Toss with oil and marjoram. Roast, turning periodically,

40 minutes until veggies are soft and beginning to brown. When eggplants are cool enough to handle, scrape out pulp into a large skillet; add remaining veggies.

3. Stir in broth. Bring to a boil over high heat. Reduce heat to medium and simmer for 35 minutes until veggies are very tender. Cool.

4. Purée soup in a blender in batches. Return soup to the saucepot. Stir in cream, salt and pepper. Heat through.

Chapter 5: Dessert Recipes

36. Keto Chocolate Caramel Pretzel Cookie Bars Recipe

37. Keto Chocolate Pecan Shortbread Drops Recipe

38. Vanilla Mousse with Rhubarb Sauce Recipe

39. Walnut Blondies Recipe

40. Strawberries with French Cream Recipe

41. Raspberry Parfait Recipe

42. Low Carb Irish Coffee Recipe

43. Atkins Pie Crust Recipe

44. Double Chocolate Pecan Ice Cream Recipe

45. Keto Coconut Thumbprints Recipe

Keto Chocolate Caramel Pretzel Cookie Bars Recipe
Prep Time: 85 Minutes
Style: American
Cook Time: 26 Minutes
Difficulty: Easy

2.7g

Protein

11.7g

Fat

3.1g

Fiber

127.8cal

Calories

INGREDIENTS

6 tablespoons butter, unsalted

1/3 cup allulose, granulated Wholesome

1 teaspoon vanilla extract

1/4 teaspoon table salt

3/4 cup almond flour, super finely ground, gluten free

2 tablespoons coconut flour, finely ground, organic

1/4 teaspoon xanthan gum

47 grams semi sweet style chocolate baking chips, 45% cocoa, no sugar added

1 bar Atkins Chocolate Caramel Pretzel Snack Bar

DIRECTIONS

1. Heat oven to 325°F. Prepare a 7 ½ by 6-inch baking dish with parchment paper.

2. In a medium bowl, blend melted butter, granulated allulose, vanilla extract and salt until completely incorporated and no clumps of sweetener remain. Add almond flour, coconut flour and xanthan gum, mixing until a thick dough develops and all flour is thoroughly incorporated. Smooth into the prepared baking dish, producing an even layer.

3. Bake for 15 minutes, then flip and bake another 10 minutes, or until golden brown on top. Watch attentively in the final 5 minutes to ensure it does not burn.

4. Remove from the oven, switch off the oven, sprinkle with chocolate chips, and put in the oven for 2 minutes, or until the chocolate chips are shiny. Allow it cool in the baking pan for 5 minutes, then use an offset spatula or rubber scraper to smooth the melted chocolate into an equal coating over the cookie. Top with coarsely diced Atkins Chocolate Caramel Pretzel Bar and sea salt flakes. Let cool another 15 minutes in the pan, then remove from the pan to cool entirely, another hour, before cutting into 12 even pieces. One piece is one serving.

Keto Chocolate Pecan Shortbread Drops Recipe

Prep Time: 20 Minutes

Style: American

Cook Time: 14 Minutes

Difficulty: Difficult

1.2g

Protein

4.9g

Fat

0.5g

Fiber

50.7cal

Calories

INGREDIENTS

- 16 tablespoons Unsalted Butter Stick
- 1/2 cup Sucralose Based Sweetener (Sugar Substitute)
- 1/2 teaspoon stevia sweetener
- 1 large Egg (Whole)
- 2 tablespoons Cream, heavy, liquid
- 1 teaspoon Vanilla Extract
- 3/4 cup(s) Soy flour, defatted (1 cup= 105g)
- 3 teaspoons Baking Powder (Straight Phosphate, Double Acting)
- 3 tablespoons Cocoa Powder
- 1/2 cup chopped Pecan Nuts

DIRECTIONS

1. Preheat the oven to 325°F.
2. With an electric mixer, whip butter, sucralose and stevia on medium speed until light and fluffy, approximately 4 minutes. Turn speed to low and add egg, cream, vanilla extract and 1 tsp chocolate extract

(optional). Scrape the bowl down, and then add soy flour, baking powder, cocoa powder and pecans, mixing until barely incorporated.

3. Drop dough by heaping teaspoonfuls onto oiled baking sheets. Bake for 12 to 14 minutes, until cookies are set. Cool on sheets 1 minute before transferring to wire racks to cool fully.

Vanilla Mousse with Rhubarb Sauce Recipe

Prep Time: 15 Minutes

Style: American

Cook Time: 10 Minutes

Difficulty: Moderate

7.3g

Protein

22.1g

Fat

1.9g

Fiber

253.7cal

Calories

INGREDIENTS

2 stalks Rhubarb

1/4 cup Tap Water

1 tablespoon Sugar Free Strawberry Jam

1/2 cup Heavy Cream

4 ounces Greek Yogurt - Plain (Container)

3 teaspoons Sucralose Based Sweetener (Sugar Substitute)

DIRECTIONS

1. For the rhubarb sauce: In a small saucepan, mix the rhubarb, water and strawberry jam; bring to a simmer over medium heat. Reduce heat to medium-low; cover and simmer, stirring periodically, until rhubarb has a sauce-like consistency, approximately 10 minutes. Set aside to cool.

2. For the vanilla mousse: In a mixing bowl, using an electric mixer on medium-high speed, whip together the cream, 4 oz yogurt, and sugar substitute to semi-firm peaks. Reserve 1/4 cup mousse for topping.

3. To assemble: Set up two martini glasses or wine glasses. Spoon 1/4 cup mousse in the bottom of each glass and distribute evenly. Top each with 1 1/2 tbsp rhubarb sauce. Divide the remaining mousse amongst the glasses, then top with the remaining rhubarb. Top with the reserved 1/4 cup mousse, dividing equally.

Walnut Blondies Recipe

Prep Time: 20 Minutes

Style: American

Cook Time: 14 Minutes

Difficulty: Difficult

8.7g

Protein

26.2g

Fat

2.1g

Fiber

286.5cal

Calories

INGREDIENTS

- 1 cup chopped English Walnuts
- 1 cup Unsalted Butter Stick
- 1 cup Sucralose Based Sweetener (Sugar Substitute)
- 1 teaspoon Vanilla Extract
- 1 cup Whole Grain Soy Flour
- 1/2 cup 100% Stone Ground Whole Wheat Pastry Flour
- 3 large Eggs (Whole)
- 1 ounce Vital Wheat Gluten
- 1 1/2 teaspoons Baking Powder (Straight Phosphate, Double Acting)
- 1/2 teaspoon Cinnamon
- 2 servings Unsweetened Baking Chocolate Squares

DIRECTIONS

1. Heat oven to 325°F. Toast walnuts on a sheet pan for 8-10 minutes, cool and then roughly chop. Set aside.

2. Line a 13-by-9-inch baking pan with aluminum foil extending 2 inches over both short edges of the pan. Grease foil, and put aside.

3. Whisk butter, sugar substitute, eggs and vanilla extract together in a large bowl. In another dish whisk flours, gluten, baking powder and cinnamon together; fold into butter mixture until thoroughly blended. Stir in walnuts. Spread evenly into the prepared pan. Bake until puffed and set, and a toothpick inserted in the middle comes out clean (top will not be browned), 12 to 14 minutes.

4. Cool fully in a pan on a wire rack. Drizzle chocolate in thin lines over the whole surface of blondies. Let stand until set, approximately 1 hour. (The recipe may be made up to this step, sealed with plastic wrap and kept at room temperature overnight.)

5. Firmly clutching the foil on both ends, remove blondies out of the pan, and set on the work surface. Cut into 12 pieces, and serve.

Strawberries with French Cream Recipe

Prep Time: 10 Minutes

Style: French

Cook Time: 0 Minutes

Difficulty: Moderate

1.5g
Protein

13.1g
Fat

1.7g
Fiber

150.4cal
Calories

INGREDIENTS

    1/2 cup Heavy Cream

    1 tablespoon Sucralose Based Sweetener (Sugar Substitute)

    3 tablespoons Sour Cream (Cultured)

    12 ounces fresh strawberries

DIRECTIONS

1. With an electric mixer on high speed, whip cream and sugar substitute until soft peaks form, approximately 4 minutes.
2. Beat in sour cream until well-mixed. Serve with berries.

Raspberry Parfait Recipe

Prep Time: 5 Minutes

Style: American

Cook Time: 0 Minutes

Difficulty: Moderate

5.6g

Protein

46.2g

Fat

2g

Fiber

464.6cal

Calories

INGREDIENTS

  1/2 cup Heavy Cream

  4 ounces Mascarpone

  2 individual packets Sucralose Based Sweetener (Sugar Substitute)

  1/2 cup Raspberries

DIRECTIONS

1. Beat 1/2 cup heavy cream until soft peaks form.

2. Add 4 oz mascarpone and 2 sachets of sweetener. Beat just till smooth. Taste and apply extra sweetness if desired.

3. Using 1/2 cup raspberries, top with the dairy mixture in 2 parfait glasses.

Low Carb Irish Coffee Recipe

Prep Time: 5 Minutes

Style: Other

Cook Time: 10 Minutes

Difficulty: Moderate

0.6g

Protein

7.3g

Fat

0g

Fiber

176 cal

Calories

INGREDIENTS

   36 fluid ounces Decaffeinated Coffee

   9 fluid ounce (no ice) Whiskey

   3 teaspoons Sucralose Based Sweetener (Sugar Substitute)

   1/2 cup Heavy Cream

DIRECTIONS

1. Brew 4 ½ cups coffee (36 fl oz) and keep warm.

2. In a small saucepan, reheat whiskey (9 fl oz= 1 cup plus 2 teaspoons) over medium-low heat (do not boil). Stir sugar replacement and warm whiskey into made coffee.

3. In the small bowl of an electric mixer, whip heavy cream on medium to soft peaks.

4. Divide coffee mixture among 6 cups (approximately 7 ½-fluid ounces, slightly short of 1 cup each serving), and top each with a dollop of whipped cream (about 2 tablespoons per serving).

Atkins Pie Crust Recipe

Prep Time: 65 Minutes

Style: American

Cook Time: 16 Minutes

Difficulty: Difficult

8.6g

Protein

13.2g

Fat

1.3g

Fiber

168.2cal

Calories

INGREDIENTS

1/3 cup 100% Stone Ground Whole Wheat Pastry Flour

1/3 cup Whole Grain Soy Flour

2 ounces Vital Wheat Gluten

3 tablespoons Plain Wheat Germ

1/2 teaspoon Salt

1/2 cup Unsalted Butter Stick

1 tablespoon Tap Water

DIRECTIONS

1. In a food processor, pulse flour, wheat gluten, germ, salt and butter until mixture forms a coarse meal. Slowly add water and continue pounding until the dough starts to come together. Turn onto a sheet of plastic wrap, roll into a ball and cover with plastic. Flatten to a 7-inch disk and refrigerate in the freezer for 15 minutes.

2. Roll dough out between 2 pieces of plastic wrap to a 12-inch circle (if required, sprinkle on 1/2 teaspoon wheat gluten flour per side to aid rolling). Remove the top piece of plastic and invert over a 9-inch pie dish. Center the dough and push against the bottom and sides of the plate. Remove plastic, roll under the edges and crimp decoratively. Chill in the freezer for 15 minutes.

3. Use unbaked crust as suggested in the recipe of your choosing. Or for a prebaked crust, preheat the oven to 400° F. Prick the bottom and corners of the pie shell with a fork. Line the pie shell with foil, fill halfway with pie weights or dry beans and flip the foil over to cover the pastry border. Bake for 16 minutes. Remove the foil and weights,

cover loosely with foil and bake a further 4 to 6 minutes or until golden. Cool on a rack for 20 minutes before using.

4. Makes 8 servings.

Double Chocolate Pecan Ice Cream Recipe

Prep Time: 300 Minutes

Style: American

Cook Time: 18 Minutes

Difficulty: Difficult

7.1g

Protein

44.3g

Fat

5.3g

Fiber

446.9cal

Calories

INGREDIENTS

1 cup chopped Pecans

1 teaspoon Gelatin Powder

1 cup Tap Water

6 large Egg Yolks

3/4 cup Sucralose Based Sweetener (Sugar Substitute)

2 1/2 cups Heavy Cream

2/3 cup Cocoa Powder (Unsweetened)

1/2 teaspoon Salt

1 1/2 teaspoons Vanilla Extract

4 tablespoons Lily's Sugar Free Chocolate Chips

DIRECTIONS

1. Preheat the oven to 350°F.

2. Toast pecans for 8 minutes, remove and let cool then cut and leave away. Sprinkle gelatin over water in a heavy bottom saucepan. Let stand until softened, approximately 5 minutes.

3. In a medium bowl, mix yolks and sugar substitute to blend. Add cream and cocoa powder to the gelatin mixture and boil over medium-low heat, stirring regularly, until chocolate is dissolved and sauce has begun to simmer.

4. Slowly add half of the gelatin mixture into the yolk mixture, stirring continuously. Pour mixture back into the pot. This technique is called tempering. Cook, stirring frequently, until mixture is thick enough to coat the back of a spoon, approximately 4 minutes. Remove from heat.

5. Stir in salt, vanilla and chocolate extracts. Chill mixture for 4 hours. Pour ice cream into the ice cream machine. Process according to manufacturer's guidelines. About 5 minutes before ice cream is completed, add pecans and chocolate.

Keto Coconut Thumbprints Recipe

Prep Time: 20 Minutes

Style: American

Cook Time: 8 Minutes

Difficulty: Difficult

1.3g

Protein

5.7g

Fat

0.7g

Fiber

60 cal

Calories

INGREDIENTS

    2/3 cup, shelled (32 kernels) Brazil Nuts

    1/2 cup Coconut, shredded, unsweetened

    1/2 cup Whole Grain Soy Flour

    2 1/2 tablespoons Sucralose Based Sweetener (Sugar Substitute)

    1/2 cup Unsalted Butter Stick

    1 large Egg (Whole)

    1 large Egg Yolk

    1 teaspoon Coconut Extract

3 tablespoons Sugar Free Seedless Blackberry Jam

DIRECTIONS

1. Preheat the oven to 375°F.
2. In a food processor, pulse 1/2 cup coconut and nuts until finely ground, approximately 1 minute. Add soy flour and sugar replacement and pulse to mix.
3. Add butter and process until mixture resembles a coarse meal, approximately 30 more seconds. Add egg, yolk and extract and pulse until dough barely comes together, approximately 1 minute.
4. Scrape dough into a basin, cover and refrigerate for at least 3 hours, until relatively stiff. Roll dough into 36 balls and lay on an ungreased baking pan. Dip your thumb into warm water and create a dip in the middle of each ball, making a doughnut-like shape (but not pressing entirely however).
5. Fill each depression with ¼ -teaspoon jam. Bake until golden, approximately 6 minutes. Cool 1 minute on a baking sheet before transferring to wire racks to cool fully.

Chapter 6: Appetizers

46. Keto Swiss Chard with Garlic Butter Recipe

47. Leeks Under Cheese Recipe

48. Zucchini Pasta with Almond Pesto Recipe

49. Tomato-Cucumber Guacamole Recipe

Keto Swiss Chard with Garlic Butter Recipe
Prep Time: 15 Minutes
Style: Other
Cook Time: 15 Minutes
Difficulty: Moderate

2.1g
Protein

4.9g
Fat

1.8g
Fiber

63.2cal

Calories

INGREDIENTS

2 pounds Swiss Chard

2 tablespoons Unsalted Butter Stick

1 tablespoon Light Olive Oil

2 teaspoons Garlic

1/2 teaspoon Salt

1/4 teaspoon Black Pepper

DIRECTIONS

1. Cut chard stems crosswise into 1/2-inch sections. Cut leaves in half lengthwise, stack them and cut crosswise into 2-inch pieces.

2. Heat butter and olive oil in a large saucepan over medium heat. Add garlic and simmer, stirring, until barely fragrant, approximately 30 seconds. Add chard stems; cover and simmer, tossing occasionally, until crisp-tender, approximately 4 minutes.

3. Add chard leaves in batches, stirring to coat; season with salt and pepper. Cover and boil, stirring once, until stems are soft and leaves are wilted, 4 to 5 minutes.

Leeks Under Cheese Recipe

Prep Time: 10 Minutes

Style: American

Cook Time: 25 Minutes

Difficulty: Moderate

7.8g

Protein

12.1g

Fat

1.6g

Fiber

188.2cal

Calories

INGREDIENTS

  1 tablespoon Unsalted Butter Stick

  1 tablespoon Canola Vegetable Oil

  4 each Leeks

  1/2 cup Chicken Broth, Bouillon or Consomme

  1/4 teaspoon Black Pepper

  1/3 cup shredded Gruyere Cheese

  1/3 cup Parmesan Cheese (Grated)

DIRECTIONS

1. In an ovenproof skillet, melt butter and oil over medium-high heat. Add chopped leeks and simmer for 5 minutes until they begin to sweat (release moisture). Add broth, salt, and pepper. Cover and continue cooking for 15 minutes until the leeks are soft. Uncover and boil off liquid in the skillet.

2. Heat broiler. Sprinkle leeks equally with cheese. Broil 3 to 4 minutes, 5 from heat source, until browned.

Zucchini Pasta with Almond Pesto Recipe

Prep Time: 10 Minutes

Style: Italian

Cook Time: 5 Minutes

Difficulty: Difficult

6g

Protein

20.1g

Fat

2.9g

Fiber

222.8cal

Calories

INGREDIENTS

   1/3 cup, whole Almonds

   1 clove Garlic

   1 cup Parsley

   1/3 cup Parmesan Cheese (Grated)

   1/3 cup Extra Virgin Olive Oil

   1 teaspoon Salt

   2 pounds Zucchini

1 tablespoon Light Olive Oil

1/8 teaspoon Crushed Red Pepper Flakes

DIRECTIONS

1. In a food processor pulse the almonds until finely ground. Add the garlic, parsley and Parmesan; pulse 4-6 times. Add in the 1/3 cup extra-virgin olive oil and 1 teaspoon salt (or to taste) and pulse again a few times. Set aside.

2. Spiralize the zucchini or use a grater with the zucchini lengthwise to produce longer strands. Preheat a large pan or wok over medium-high heat with 1 tablespoon olive oil. Cook the zucchini for 4 minutes using tongs to toss and rotate until cooked through, approximately 5 minutes.

3. Toss the heated zucchini with the pesto, sprinkle with the crushed red chili pepper flakes (optional) and divide into spaghetti bowls. Season with extra salt and pepper to taste. Serve immediately.

4. Note: to roast raw almonds, heat oven to 350°F, scatter nuts on a sheet pan and bake for 10 minutes. Cool before using.

Tomato-Cucumber Guacamole Recipe

Prep Time: 15 Minutes

Style: Mexican

Cook Time: 0 Minutes

Difficulty: Moderate

1.5g

Protein

6.8g

Fat

3.8g

Fiber

87.8cal

Calories

INGREDIENTS

    2 medium whole (2-3/5" diameter) Red Tomatoes

    2 medium Cucumber (Peeled)

    2 fruit without skin and seeds California Avocados

    1/4 cup chopped Red Onions

    1 1/2 fluid ounces Fresh Lime Juice

    1/2 teaspoon Cumin

DIRECTIONS

1. Dice the tomatoes, cucumber, avocado and onions. Juice and zest the lime.
2. In a medium bowl, gently combine tomatoes, cucumbers, avocados, onion, 3 Tbsp lime juice, 1 tsp lime zest and cumin.
3. Season to taste with salt and pepper.

Chapter 7: Side Dishes and Snacks

61. Low Carb Ranch Fried String Cheese Recipe

62. Carrot-Nut Muffins Recipe

63. Vegetarian "Ham," Cream Cheese and Dill Pickle Roll-Ups Recipe

64. Keto Zucchini Bread Muffins Recipe

65. Cherry Hazelnut Biscotti Recipe

66. Sautéed Cocktail Meatballs Recipe

67. Keto Sweet and Salty Almonds Recipe

68. Chili Spiced Tortilla Wraps Recipe

69. Cardamom Butter Cookies Recipe

70. Keto Sweet and Spicy Nuts Recipe

Orange-Spiced Sweet Potato Pancakes Recipe

Prep Time: 15 Minutes

Style: American

Cook Time: 15 Minutes

Difficulty: Moderate

7g

Protein

11.2g

Fat

2.7g

Fiber

176 cal

Calories

INGREDIENTS

1 pound Sweet Potato

1/3 serving Atkins Soy-Free Flour Mix

1 small Onion

2 large Eggs (Whole)

3 teaspoons Orange Zest

1 teaspoon Salt

1/2 teaspoon Cinnamon

6 tablespoons canola oil

DIRECTIONS

1. Peel and shred sweet potatoes on a grater. Combine sweet potatoes, sliced onion, 1/3 cup flour mix, eggs, orange zest, salt, and cinnamon in a large basin.

2. Heat ¼ cup oil in a large pan over medium-high heat. Drop 2-tablespoon mounds of sweet potato mixture into pan, flattening slightly; cook in batches until golden brown, approximately 2 minutes each side. Drain on paper towels and serve hot. Add remaining 2 tablespoons of oil after 3 batches.

3. This recipe produces around 20 pancakes; each serving is two pancakes.

Broccoli Rabe Parmigiano Recipe

Prep Time: 15 Minutes

Style: Italian

Cook Time: 10 Minutes

Difficulty: Moderate

8.1g

Protein

7.6g

Fat

3.9g

Fiber

112.4cal

Calories

INGREDIENTS

2 tablespoons Extra Virgin Olive Oil

2 cloves Garlic

1/4 teaspoon Crushed Red Pepper Flakes

2 pounds fresh broccoli rabe

1/4 cup Tap Water

2 tablespoons Fresh Lemon Juice

2 teaspoons Lemon Zest

1/8 teaspoon Salt

1/8 teaspoon Black Pepper

1/2 cup Parmesan Cheese (Grated)

DIRECTIONS

1. Broccoli rabe has stalks that range in length from six to nine inches and clusters of small buds that resemble broccoli. It has a flavor that is more astringent than that of its more well-known relative. In either sautéing or braising, it is a wonderful preparation. If you would rather not use broccoli in this dish, you are welcome to do so any time. chop a head of broccoli that weighs two pounds into little florets, then remove the stalks and chop them into pieces that are half an inch in size.

2. Oil should be heated over medium-high heat in a big pan with a deep well. Stir in the pepper flakes and minced garlic, then sauté for thirty seconds.

3. Add broccoli rabe, water, lemon juice and lemon zest; stir well. Cover the pan and cook the broccoli rabe over medium heat for eight minutes, or until it reaches a crisp-tender consistency.

4. Salt and freshly ground black pepper should be used to season the food to taste.

5. On a serving plate, transfer the mixture, and then sprinkle it with Parmesan.

Ratatouille Recipe

Prep Time: 30 Minutes

Style: French

Cook Time: 45 Minutes

Difficulty: Difficult

2.2g

Protein

12.3g

Fat

4.6g

Fiber

150.8cal

Calories

INGREDIENTS

1 eggplant, unpeeled (approx 1-1/4 lb) Eggplant

1/3 cup Extra Virgin Olive Oil

2 teaspoons Garlic

1 medium Zucchini

1 teaspoon Salt

1/2 teaspoon Rosemary (Dried)

1/2 tablespoon leaf Thyme (Dried)

1/4 teaspoon Black Pepper

1 small Onion

1 small Sweet Red Pepper

1 small whole (2-2/5" diameter) Red Tomato

1 medium Yellow Summer Squash

DIRECTIONS

1. Sprinkle eggplant with salt; set in a strainer and allow bitter juices to drain for 20 minutes. Rinse eggplant and pat dry.

2. Heat oven to 425°F. In a 10x15 baking dish, combine oil, minced garlic, salt, rosemary, thyme, and pepper. Evenly dice all the veggies including eggplant and then put together in the baking dish with the oil mixture.

3. Cover the dish with foil and bake for 15 minutes. Uncover and cook 30 minutes longer, tossing periodically, until veggies are soft and browned.

Cauliflower-Leek Puree Recipe

Prep Time: 10 Minutes

Style: American

Cook Time: 15 Minutes

Difficulty: Moderate

1.4g
Protein

8.6g

Fat

1.5g

Fiber

98.4cal

Calories

INGREDIENTS

3 cups Cauliflower

1 each Leek

3 tablespoons Unsalted Butter Stick

3 tablespoons Heavy Cream

1/8 teaspoon Nutmeg (Ground)

DIRECTIONS

1. Cook chopped cauliflower and sliced leeks in mildly salted (approximately 1 tsp) boiling water for 15 minutes, until very soft. Drain; return vegetables to saucepan and stir in pan over high heat to fully evaporate extra liquid.

2. Place half the veggies in the food processor with half the butter and cream. Process till smooth. Repeat with remaining veggies, butter, and cream.

3. Mix in nutmeg (optional); season to taste with salt and pepper.

Keto Egg Drop Soup Recipe

Prep Time: 5 Minutes

Style: Asian

Cook Time: 10 Minutes

Difficulty: Moderate

7.7g
Protein

4.3g
Fat

0.2g
Fiber

79.4cal
Calories

INGREDIENTS

    2 14.5 ounces cans Chicken Broth, Bouillon or Consomme

    1 teaspoon Ginger

    2 large Eggs (Whole)

    2 medium (4-1/8" long) Scallions or Spring Onions

    1/2 teaspoon Toasted Sesame Oil

DIRECTIONS

1. In a medium saucepan over high heat, bring broth and minced ginger to a boil. Turn heat down to a simmer and gently pour in egg to produce golden threads.

2. Turn heat off and add chopped green onions, sesame oil and soy sauce to taste. Serve immediately.

Cauliflower and Onion Mash with Cheddar Recipe

Prep Time: 5 Minutes

Style: American

Cook Time: 8 Minutes

Difficulty: Moderate

8.3g

Protein

13.9g

Fat

1.7g

Fiber

178.7cal

Calories

INGREDIENTS

1/2 cup Cauliflower

1 teaspoon Extra Virgin Olive Oil

3 tablespoons chopped Onions

1/4 cup shredded Cheddar Cheese

DIRECTIONS
1. Steam cauliflower in a steamer basket over boiling water until tender, approximately 3-4 minutes. Mash with a fork.
2. Meanwhile, heat a nonstick pan with 1 teaspoon of virgin olive oil over medium-high heat. Add onions and sauté until tender.
3. Add onions to mashed cauliflower and top with cheese.

Wild Rice, Sausage and Cherry Stuffing Recipe

Prep Time: 60 Minutes

Style: American

Cook Time: 45 Minutes

Difficulty: Difficult

11.3g
Protein

16.6g
Fat

1.7g
Fiber

235.1cal

Calories

INGREDIENTS

3/4 cup chopped Onions

4 servings Atkins Low Carb Wheat Bread

1/3 cup Wild Rice

2 1/2 cups Tap Water

12 ounce raw (yield after cooking) Italian Sausage

1/4 cup Unsalted Butter Stick

3 stalk, medium (7-1/2" - 8" long) Celery

1/2 cup Parsley

1/3 cup, with pits, yield Red Sour Cherries

1 tablespoon Poultry Seasoning

1/2 teaspoon Black Pepper

1 cup Chicken Broth, Bouillon or Consomme

DIRECTIONS

1. Combine wild rice, 1 1/2 cups of the water and a liberal amount of salt in a small saucepan; bring to a boil over high heat. Reduce heat to medium, cover and simmer until tender, 40 to 45 minutes. Drain and put aside.

2. Heat oven to 350°F. Set bread cubes on a jelly-roll pan in a single layer. Bake, tossing once, until crispy, 10 to 14 minutes. Transfer to a big bowl.

3. Meanwhile, take sausage from casing; crumble into a large nonstick pan over medium heat. Cook, tossing regularly to break up clumps, until cooked through and gently browned, approximately 12 minutes. Add to bread.

4. Return skillet to medium heat; add butter. When melted, add celery and white onion; simmer, stirring regularly, until soft, approximately 10 minutes.

5. Add to bread mixture, then whisk in parsley, cherries, poultry seasoning, pepper and wild rice. Mix thoroughly. Stir in 1 cup of the chicken stock; add more if the stuffing still appears dry.

6. Transfer the filling to a large baking dish. Cover with foil and bake for 30 minutes, then uncover and continue baking until gently browned and cooked through, 15 minutes more.

Atkins Cornbread Recipe

Prep Time: 10 Minutes

Style: American

Cook Time: 30 Minutes

Difficulty: Difficult

8.6g

Protein

12.7g

Fat

0.5g

Fiber

154.4cal

Calories

INGREDIENTS

3 large Eggs

1 cup Whole Milk

1/3 cup Vegetable Oil

2 tablespoons Unsalted Butter Stick

8 ounces Monterey Jack Cheese with Jalapeno

1 each Chipotle en Adobo, whole

1/2 cup Whole Grain Soy Flour

2 ounces Vital Wheat Gluten

3 teaspoons Baking Powder (Sodium Aluminum Sulfate, Double Acting)

DIRECTIONS
1. Preheat the oven to 350°F.
2. Mist an 8-inch square baking pan with olive oil spray.

3. In a medium bowl, beat egg, milk, oil and melted butter. Shred the cheeses and cut the chilies, add them and mix until thoroughly integrated.

4. Add soy flour, wheat gluten (1/4 cup) and baking powder, whisking until ingredients are just incorporated (batter will be stiff). Spread mixture into prepared pan. Bake until golden.

5. Cool on a wire rack 5 to 10 minutes before cutting into 16 servings (2x2-inch squares).

Buffalo Hot Wing Cauliflower Recipe
Prep Time: 10 Minutes
Style: American
Cook Time: 40 Minutes
Difficulty: Moderate

6.5g
Protein

12.4g
Fat

5.3g
Fiber

175.4cal
Calories

INGREDIENTS

1 head large (6-7" diameter) Cauliflower

1 tablespoon Olive Oil

4 tablespoons Red Hot Buffalo Wing Sauce

3 teaspoons Sriracha Hot Chili Sauce

2 tablespoons Unsalted Butter Stick

1 1/3 tablespoons Apple Cider Vinegar

1 1/2 ounces Blue or Roquefort Cheese

DIRECTIONS

1. Preheat the oven to 375°F.

2. Cut the cauliflower into small florets and sprinkle with the olive oil. Roast on a baking sheet for 35-40 minutes, or until tender.

3. When cauliflower has approximately 10 minutes remaining to roast, heat a large pan over medium heat. Add the hot wing sauce and Sriracha to the skillet and simmer until sizzling and reduced to a paste, approximately 5 minutes. Remove from heat and mix in the butter and vinegar.

4. When the cauliflower is done roasting, return it to the pan with the sauce and stir to evenly cover all the cauliflower. Serve immediately with blue cheese sprinkled over top.

Keto Herb-Butter Blend Recipe

Prep Time: 7 Minutes

Style: American

Cook Time: 0 Minutes

Difficulty: Moderate

0.1g
Protein

12.5g
Fat

0.1g
Fiber

110.7cal
Calories

INGREDIENTS

   1/2 teaspoon Salt

   1 teaspoon Black Pepper

   1/2 cup Extra Virgin Olive Oil

   1 teaspoon Garlic

   3 teaspoons leaves Oregano

   2 tablespoons Basil

   1 cup Unsalted Butter Stick

   1/2 cup Coconut Oil

DIRECTIONS

This flavorful butter is great on veggies, seafood and meats. Each serving is 1 Tbsp.

1. Place salt, pepper, olive oil, garlic, oregano and basil in a food processor. Pulse until herbs are finely minced and there are no visible particles of pepper (30-60 seconds total).
2. Add butter and coconut oil, mixing until smooth.
3. Scrape into a jar with a snap cover and refrigerate up to 1 month.

Broccoli and Cauliflower with Vegan "Cheese" Sauce Recipe

Prep Time: 15 Minutes

Style: Other

Cook Time: 15 Minutes

Difficulty: Difficult

8.3g
Protein

11.3g
Fat

5.1g
Fiber

190.4cal
Calories

INGREDIENTS

2 cup florets Broccoli Flower Clusters

2 cups Cauliflower

3 tablespoons Olive Oil

1/2 cup chopped Onions

2 cloves Garlic

1 cup Organic Vegetable Broth

3 servings Nutritional Yeast

1/8 teaspoon Red or Cayenne Pepper

1/2 teaspoon Salt

1/4 teaspoon Black Pepper

1/4 teaspoon Turmeric (Ground)

1 1/2 tablespoons Spelt Flour

1/2 cup chopped Red Sweet Pepper

1/4 cup chopped Scallions or Spring Onions

DIRECTIONS

1. The essence of vegan comfort food, this side dish adds nutritional yeast, available at natural foods shops, to provide cheese-like taste, and almonds to this delightful vegetable mix. Nutritional yeast is an excellent source of protein and B-vitamins. Although it's optional, the turmeric provides the sauce lovely golden tint, evoking Cheddar cheese. Serve with Walnut-Crusted Tofu Cutlets.

2. Fill a medium saucepan with 1½ inches of water; insert a steamer basket and add the broccoli and cauliflower. Cover and bring to a boil over high heat. Reduce the heat to medium and steam until the veggies are barely tender, about 7 minutes.

3. Meanwhile, add 1 tablespoon of olive oil to a small sauté pan over medium-high heat and cook for 30 seconds. Add the onion and minced garlic and heat until the onions are transparent, roughly 3 minutes, stirring often.

4. Reduce the heat to medium and add the broth, nutritional yeast, cayenne, salt, ground pepper and turmeric (if using) and mix well.

5. Using a fork or tiny whisk, put the remaining 2 tablespoons of olive oil as well as the flour in a small bowl and stir thoroughly, being careful to remove any lumps. Add to the sauté pan, combine well and simmer until the sauce thickens, stirring periodically, about 2 minutes. Remove from the heat.

6. When the broccoli and cauliflower are done, arrange them on a serving dish. Top the veggies with the sauce and garnish with sliced bell pepper and scallions.

DIRECTIONS

1. Broccoli and Cauliflower with Vegan "Cheese" Sauce and Herbs Stir a tablespoon of fresh minced herbs such as basil, parsley or dill into the sauce after cooking.

2. Mixed Vegetable Medley Follow the basic recipe, substituting the broccoli and cauliflower with an equal number of non starchy vegetables such as zucchini, cabbage, fennel, broccoli rabe, celery and/or bok choy.

Low Carb Ranch Fried String Cheese Recipe

Prep Time: 35 Minutes

Style: American

Cook Time: 4 Minutes

Difficulty: Moderate

10.9g

Protein

6.8g

Fat

0.9g

Fiber

167.7cal

Calories

INGREDIENTS

5 eas string mozzarella cheese

1 tablespoon almond flour, super finely ground, gluten free

1 lrg raw egg

1/2 tablespoon tap water

1 bag Atkins Ranch Protein Chips

4 teaspoons olive oil

1 teaspoon fresh young green scallions, chopped

DIRECTIONS

1. Cut string cheese in half. In one of three shallow dishes, put the almond flour. In the next bowl, mix together the egg and water. In the final bowl, put crumbled Atkins Ranch Protein Chips. Working one at a time, gently coat each piece of string cheese with almond flour, then dip in the egg mix to coat and then coat in crumbled chips. Place each coated string cheese on a dish and freeze for 30 minutes.

2. Heat air fryer to 375°F for at least 3 minutes.

3. Remove cheese sticks from the freezer and liberally cover with olive oil spray. Place in a single layer in the air fryer and cook for 3-4 minutes, until the cheese is melted and the coating is brown but not scorching.

4. Remove from the air fryer and serve garnished with scallion while warm. Each serving is two cheese sticks.

Carrot-Nut Muffins Recipe

Prep Time: 10 Minutes

Style: Other

Cook Time: 25 Minutes

Difficulty: Difficult

8.5g

Protein

21.4g

Fat

2.2g

Fiber

239.6cal

Calories

INGREDIENTS

1 cup almond flour, super finely ground, gluten free

1 cup Magic Baker zero sugar baking blend, Splenda

2 scoops multi purpose protein powder, gluten free

1/4 cup coconut flour, finely ground, organic

2 teaspoons cinnamon, ground

1/2 teaspoon table salt

1/2 teaspoon baking powder, low sodium

1 cup fresh carrots, grated

3/4 cup canola oil

4 lrgs raw egg

2 teaspoons vanilla extract

DIRECTIONS

1. *Ingredient note:* Look for a whey protein powder with 1 gram or fewer net carbohydrates per ounce, and use 2 1-ounce scoops for this recipe.

2. Preheat the oven to 350°F. Prepare 12 muffin pan wells with paper liners, or gently grease.

3. In a large bowl mix together almond flour, no sugar sweetener, whey protein powder, coconut flour, cinnamon, salt and baking powder until no clumps remain.

4. In a medium bowl, mix together grated carrot, vegetable oil, room temperature eggs, and vanilla extract. Pour carrot mixture into flour mixture. Stir until just mixed. Pour around ¼ cup batter into each ready muffin well..

5. Bake for 25-30 minutes until golden brown, and a cake tester inserted in the center comes out clean. Cool on a wire rack. One muffin as indicated is one serving.

Vegetarian "Ham," Cream Cheese and Dill Pickle Roll-Ups Recipe

Prep Time: 5 Minutes

Style: American

Cook Time: 0 Minutes

Difficulty: Moderate

21g

Protein

11.9g

Fat

1.6g

Fiber

229.6cal

Calories

INGREDIENTS

1 1/2 servings Smart Deli Baked Ham Style

2 tablespoons Cream Cheese

2 medium Pickles

DIRECTIONS

1. Layer 3 slices of ham, spread 1 tablespoon cream cheese over the layers.
2. Place 1 pickle spear at one end and roll-up. Pin with a toothpick if desired.
3. Repeat for remaining ham, cream cheese and pickle spear.

Keto Zucchini Bread Muffins Recipe

Prep Time: 10 Minutes

Style: American

Cook Time: 25 Minutes

Difficulty: Difficult

10.3g

Protein

12.4g

Fat

5.9g

Fiber

174.8cal

Calories

INGREDIENTS

2 large Eggs (Whole)

2 tablespoons Canola Vegetable Oil

1 teaspoon Vanilla Extract

4 1/2 ounces Zucchini

1 cup Organic 100% Whole Ground Golden Flaxseed Meal

1 ounce Vanilla Whey Protein

1/3 cup Sucralose Based Sweetener (Sugar Substitute)

1 1/2 teaspoons Cinnamon

3/4 teaspoon Baking Powder (Straight Phosphate, Double Acting)

1/4 teaspoon Salt

1/8 teaspoon Allspice Ground

1/8 teaspoon Nutmeg (Ground)

DIRECTIONS

1. Preheat an oven to 350°F. Grease 6 wells of a regular non-stick muffin tray.

2. Combine the eggs, oil and vanilla in a small bowl. Using a whisk, beat until foamy for approximately 1 minute. Shred the zucchini, add it to the bowl mixing to blend.

3. Add the flax meal, protein powder, granular sugar replacement, baking powder, salt, and spices. Mix with a spoon to mix.

4. Bake for 25 minutes until slightly puffed, golden and cooked through. Enjoy with cream cheese if preferred.

Cherry Hazelnut Biscotti Recipe

Prep Time: 45 Minutes

Style: Italian

Cook Time: 73 Minutes

Difficulty: Moderate

4.2g

Protein

13.9g

Fat

2.1g

Fiber

157.9cal

Calories

INGREDIENTS

1 1/2 cups hazelnuts, chopped

1 cup almond flour, super finely ground, gluten free

1/3 cup sucralose artificial sweetener, granular

2 tablespoons coconut flour, finely ground, organic

1/2 teaspoon cinnamon, ground

1/4 teaspoon table salt

2 lrgs raw egg

3 tablespoons butter, unsalted

2 tablespoons sour cream

1/4 cup dried cherries, organic, unsweetened

DIRECTIONS

1. Heat oven to 350°F. Line a baking sheet with parchment paper.
2. Finely chop 1 cup of the hazelnuts (save 1/2 cup of coarsely chopped hazelnuts). Place in a large bowl and stir together with the almond flour, granulated sugar, coconut flour, ground cinnamon and salt. Add eggs, melted butter, and sour cream and whisk until thoroughly blended. Dough will be sticky and thick. Fold in chopped cherries and remaining ½ cup coarsely chopped hazelnuts.
3. On a prepared baking sheet, shape dough into a log; ¾-inch high, 4-inches broad and 8-inches long. Bake for 25-30 minutes, till golden brown. Transfer to a wire rack to cool for 30 minutes.
4. Reduce oven temperature to 300°F. Carefully cut logs crosswise, using a serrated knife, into 16, ½-inch broad slices. Arrange slices on a baking sheet and bake for 9 minutes. Flip and cook 9-15 minutes longer, until bottoms are beautifully browned. Turn off the oven and set a wooden spoon in the door to hold it open, allowing the biscotti to cool gently and crisp for at least another 30 minutes. One piece of biscotti is one serving.

Sautéed Cocktail Meatballs Recipe

Prep Time: 10 Minutes

Style: Mediterranean/Greek

Cook Time: 20 Minutes

Difficulty: Difficult

40.5g

Protein

32.8g

Fat

1.8g

Fiber

476.7cal

Calories

INGREDIENTS

- 1/2 cup Blanched Almond Flour
- 1/2 pound Ground Beef (90% Lean / 10% Fat)
- 1/2 pound Ground Pork
- 1/2 pound Ground Veal

1/4 cup Parmesan Cheese (Grated)

2 large Eggs (Whole)

1/4 cup sprig Dill

1/2 teaspoon Garlic

1 tablespoon Peppermint (Mint)

1/2 teaspoon leaf Oregano

1/4 teaspoon Cinnamon

1 tablespoon Salt

1/2 teaspoon Black Pepper

DIRECTIONS

1. Combine almond meal, meats, cheese, eggs, dill, minced garlic, mint, oregano, cinnamon, salt, and pepper; mix gently with your hands.

2. Moisten your hands (this helps keep mixture from sticking); form mixture into 1-inch balls and leave aside.

3. Place 2 tablespoons of olive oil in a large nonstick pan over medium-high heat. Add half the meatballs; cook, flipping often until browned on both sides and cooked through, approximately 8 minutes. Repeat with 2 more tablespoons of olive oil and remaining meatballs. Serve with toothpicks or wooden skewers as an appetizer.

Keto Sweet and Salty Almonds Recipe

Prep Time: 5 Minutes

Style: American

Cook Time: 15 Minutes

Difficulty: Moderate

4g

Protein

9.1g

Fat

2.3g

Fiber

106.8cal

Calories

INGREDIENTS

1 large Egg White

1/3 cup Sucralose Based Sweetener (Sugar Substitute)

3/4 dash Salt

2 teaspoons Cinnamon

2 cup, wholes Almonds

DIRECTIONS
1. Heat oven to 350°F.

2. Combine the egg white, sugar substitute, salt, and cinnamon in a medium bowl. Beat with a fork until foamy. Add almonds and toss to coat. Spread out in a single layer on a nonstick baking sheet or a baking sheet coated with aluminum foil.

3. Bake for 12-15 minutes, rotating once, until toasted and crisp. Remove from the oven and set the baking sheet on a baking rack. When the nuts are cold, remove from the pan and store in an airtight container at room temperature up to one week.

Cardamom Butter Cookies Recipe
Prep Time: 45 Minutes
Style: American
Cook Time: 10 Minutes
Phase: Phase 3
Difficulty: Moderate

3.8g

Protein

7g

Fat

0.9g

Fiber

86 cal

Calories

INGREDIENTS

1 1/2 servings Atkins Soy-Free Flour Mix

1/2 cup Blanched Almond Flour

1/4 teaspoon Baking Powder (Straight Phosphate, Double Acting)

1/2 teaspoon Salt

10 tablespoons Unsalted Butter Stick

1/2 cup Sucralose Based Sweetener (Sugar Substitute)

1 large Egg (Whole)

1 tablespoon Tap Water

2 teaspoons Vanilla Extract

1 teaspoon confectioners erythritol sweetener

3/4 tsp, ground Cardamom

8 teaspoons tap water

1/8 teaspoon cardamom, ground

DIRECTIONS
1. Please use the Atkins recipe for Atkins Soy-Free Flour Mix sweet version with vanilla whey protein for this dish. For this dish you will need 1 1/2 cups of the mix (1 1/2 serves, or half a recipe). If you modify the serving size for the recipe to boost or reduce it you will need to adapt proportionately.

2. Combine Atkins Soy-Free Flour Mix, almond flour, baking powder, and salt in a medium bowl.

3. In the large bowl of a stand mixer, whip together room temperature butter and sugar substitute until light and fluffy. Add room temperature egg, water, vanilla, and ¾ teaspoon cardamom; beat on medium speed until mixed, scraping down sides of bowl as required (mixture may seem watery). Add flour mixture a little bit at a time, mixing on low speed until dough comes together.

4. Wrap dough in parchment paper, put in a resealable bag and chill in the refrigerator for 30 minutes.

5. Heat oven to 350°F. Line 2 baking pans with parchment paper.

6. Roll dough out between paper to ¼-inch thick; use tiny cookie cutters or a sharp knife to cut out designs. If the dough is too sticky, or is not retaining the forms properly, put rolled out dough in the freezer for 10 minutes and try again. You should have roughly 50 (9-gram raw

dough apiece) cookies. Bake for 10 minutes, or until bottoms are brown, watching attentively in the final five minutes to ensure they do not burn. Cool on baking pans for 5 minutes, then remove cookies to a wire rack to cool fully.

7. While the cookies are cooling, in a separate bowl mix the confectioners erythritol, 8 tablespoons water and 1/8 teaspoon cardamom with a fork until a paste forms. Drizzle cooled cookies evenly with frosting and let dry before storing.

8. Store in an airtight container for up to 1 week. Two cookies (or 14 g cooked dough) is one serving.

Chili Spiced Tortilla Wraps Recipe
Prep Time: 5 Minutes

Style: American

Cook Time: 15 Minutes

Difficulty: Difficult

4.5g

Protein

4.3g

Fat

2.5g

Fiber

73.7cal

Calories

INGREDIENTS

    3 tablespoons Organic High Fiber Coconut Flour

    3/4 teaspoon Chili Powder

    1 tablespoon Organic 100% Whole Ground Golden Flaxseed Meal

    1/8 teaspoon Salt

    1/2 cup Coconut Milk Unsweetened

    2 whites Egg White

    1 each Egg

    1/2 teaspoon Xylitol

    1 teaspoon Olive Oil

DIRECTIONS

1. Combine coconut flour, chili powder, flax meal, and salt in a small bowl. Set aside.

2. Whisk the egg whites, whole egg, coconut milk, and sugar replacement. Add the flour mixture, whisk to blend, then leave it set for 5 minutes.

3. Preheat an electric griddle to 350°F. Lightly brush the skillet with oil. Measure ¼ cup of batter onto the griddle, spreading out into a 5-inch tortilla shape, no more than 1/4 –inch thick. Cook for at least 7 minutes on the first side, until it can be turned with a spatula without coming apart. Flip and cook for another 3 minutes, or until cooked through and beginning to brown on the edges. Repeat, brushing with oil between batches, until 4 tortilla wraps are created.

4. Place cooked tortillas on a paper towel with a paper towel between each. Eat while warm, or refrigerate for up to a week in an airtight container with paper towels between. Warm in a dry skillet over medium high for 30 seconds each side before serving. Alternatively, freeze for up to 3 months. One tortilla is one serving.

No electric griddle? These may be prepared on the stove top. Heat a large non-stick pan with 1 teaspoon of oil over medium-high heat. Reduce heat to medium, and using a 1/4 cup measure, pour batter into pan and spread out into a 5-inch tortilla shape. Allow to cook for 3-5 minutes, until golden brown below and thoroughly set on the top. Flip over and cook 1-3 more minutes. Repeat for the remaining 3 tortillas.

Keto Sweet and Spicy Nuts Recipe
Prep Time: 10 Minutes

Style: Other

Cook Time: 50 Minutes

Difficulty: Moderate

4.6g

Protein

19.4g

Fat

2.9g

Fiber

199.5cal

Calories

INGREDIENTS

1 large Egg White

1 fluid ounce Tap Water

2 tablespoons Sucralose Based Sweetener (Sugar Substitute)

1/4 teaspoon Salt

1/4 teaspoon Black Pepper

1/4 teaspoon Cumin

1/4 teaspoon Cinnamon

1/8 teaspoon Red or Cayenne Pepper

1/2 cup, half Pecan Nuts

1/2 cup, whole Almonds

1/2 cup shelled (50 halves) English Walnuts

1/2 cup, whole or half Macadamia Nuts

DIRECTIONS
1. Heat oven to 275°F. Line a baking sheet with aluminum foil; coat with nonstick cooking spray.
2. In a large bowl, combine egg white, water, sugar replacement, salt, pepper, cumin, cinnamon and 1/8 tsp cayenne (or to taste). Add nuts; stir until evenly coated.
3. Spread nuts in a single layer on a prepared baking sheet. Bake for 50 minutes to 1 hour until golden brown.

Chapter 8: Smoothie Recipes

71. Vegan Keto Coconut Protein Shake Recipe

72. Low Carb Irish Coffee Recipe

73. Almond Raspberry Smoothie Recipe

74. Keto Iced Chamomile Tea Recipe

75. Rhuberry Margarita Recipe

76. Raspberry Soy Frappe Recipe

77. Lovers' Flutes Recipe

Vegan Keto Coconut Protein Shake Recipe
Prep Time: 5 Minutes
Style: American
Cook Time: 0 Minutes
Difficulty: Moderate

24.4g
Protein

5.6g
Fat

1g
Fiber

158.7cal

Calories

INGREDIENTS

1 cup Coconut Milk Unsweetened

1 ounce Protein Technologies International ProPlus Soy Protein Isolate

1/2 teaspoon Vanilla Extract

DIRECTIONS

Whey protein powder may be substituted (please add 1g NC additional to the total NC value) for non-vegans or vegetarians.

1. Combine all ingredients in a blender with 2-4 ice cubes (depending upon the thickness desired). Consider adding coconut extract in addition to or instead of the vanilla.
2. Blend thoroughly and enjoy.

Low Carb Irish Coffee Recipe

Prep Time: 5 Minutes

Style: Other

Cook Time: 10 Minutes

Difficulty: Moderate

0.6g

Protein

7.3g
Fat

0g
Fiber

176 cal
Calories

INGREDIENTS

36 fluid ounces Decaffeinated Coffee

9 fluid ounce (no ice) Whiskey

3 teaspoons Sucralose Based Sweetener (Sugar Substitute)

1/2 cup Heavy Cream

DIRECTIONS

1. Brew 4 ½ cups coffee (36 fl oz) and keep warm.

2. In a small saucepan, reheat whiskey (9 fl oz= 1 cup plus 2 teaspoons) over medium-low heat (do not boil). Stir sugar replacement and warm whiskey into made coffee.

3. In the small bowl of an electric mixer, whip heavy cream on medium to soft peaks.

4. Divide coffee mixture among 6 cups (approximately 7 ½-fluid ounces, slightly short of 1 cup each serving), and top each with a dollop of whipped cream (about 2 tablespoons per serving).

Almond Raspberry Smoothie Recipe

Prep Time: 5 Minutes

Style: American

Cook Time: 0 Minutes

Difficulty: Moderate

18.2g

Protein

13.7g

Fat

6.9g

Fiber

259.4cal

Calories

INGREDIENTS

   4 ounces Greek Yogurt - Plain (Container)

   1/2 cup Red Raspberries

   20 each wholes Blanched & Slivered Almonds

   1/2 cup Pure Almond Milk - Unsweetened Original

DIRECTIONS

1. Feel free to come up with your own mix of various berries and nuts for this protein-packed smoothie. If you use frozen raspberries, make sure they include no added sugar.

2. Combine the yogurt, raspberries, almonds and almond milk in a blender and purée until smooth and creamy.

Keto Iced Chamomile Tea Recipe

Prep Time: 60 Minutes

Style: Other

Cook Time: 0 Minutes

Difficulty: Moderate

0g
Protein

0g
Fat

0g
Fibcr

1.3cal
Calories

INGREDIENTS

6 servings Tea, Chamomile, Bigelow Herb Tea (1 tea bag)

6 cups Tap Water

1 teaspoon No Calorie Sweetener

1 fluid ounce Fresh Lemon Juice

DIRECTIONS

Drinking naturally keto and low carb chamomile tea, particularly over ice, is a delightful approach to help strengthen your immune system and enhance metabolism.

1. Brew tea bags in water for 10 minutes. Chill 1 hour.

2. Dissolve sugar substitute in cold tea.

3. Add lemon juice. Serve over ice.

Rhuberry Margarita Recipe

Prep Time: 5 Minutes

Style: American

Cook Time: 0 Minutes

Difficulty: Moderate

0.4g
Protein

0.1g
Fat

3.4g
Fiber

85.8cal

Calories

INGREDIENTS

1 serving Keto Strawberry Rhubarb Sauce

1 1/2 tablespoons Fresh Lime Juice

1 teaspoon Sweetener

1 fluid ounce (no ice) Tequila

4 ice cubes Tap Water

2 fluid ounces Club Soda

DIRECTIONS

1. Use the Atkins recipe to create Strawberry Rhubarb Sauce for this dish. You will need 2 teaspoons for each serving. Truvia is the suggested sweetener (if using sucralose use 4 tsp and add 2g NC to the total).

2. Combine 2 tablespoons of Strawberry Rhubarb Sauce with the lime juice, sugar substitute and tequila in a blender. Pulse 2-3 times to purée the sauce.

3. Add 4 ice cubes to a glass, pour the tequila mixture over the top and add club soda or seltzer. Or make it frozen by putting it together in a blender.

Raspberry Soy Frappe Recipe

Prep Time: 5 Minutes

Style: American

Cook Time: 0 Minutes

Difficulty: Moderate

8.5g

Protein

4.8g

Fat

10.1g

Fiber

148 cal

Calories

INGREDIENTS

 - 1/2 cup Unsweetened Frozen Raspberries
 - 1 cup Organic Unsweetened Soy Milk
 - 2 packets No Calorie Sweetener Packets
 - 1/4 teaspoon Pure Almond Extract

DIRECTIONS

1. Blend all items on high until smooth.
2. Add 1/2-cup of crushed ice (or 3 ice cubes) and mix again until smooth. Enjoy!

Lovers' Flutes Recipe

Prep Time: 5 Minutes

Style: American

Cook Time: 0 Minutes

Difficulty: Moderate

0g
Protein

0g
Fat

0.2g
Fiber

113.5cal
Calories

INGREDIENTS

  1 teaspoon No Calorie Sweetener

  2/3 fluid ounce (no ice) Vodka

  1/4 fluid ounce Red Table Wine

  2 teaspoons Orange Peel

  8 ounces Champagne, Brut, Andre

DIRECTIONS

For this dish, if available, replace Campari for the red wine and use a dry champagne or a dry sparkling white wine.

1. In a cup, whisk granulated sugar substitute (according to your liking) with vodka until dissolved.

2. Evenly split the vodka and 2 tsp Campari into 2 champagne glasses. Twist the orange peel, then drop into glasses.

3. Tipping glasses slightly, gently pour in champagne down the edge of each glass. Serve immediately.

Chapter 9: Salad Recipes

78. Tabbouleh Salad Recipe

79. Mediterranean Vegetable and Egg Salad Recipe

80. Keto Caprese Salad Recipe

81. Italian Chopped Salad Recipe

82. Grilled Chicken over Baby Spinach, Tomato and Avocado Salad Recipe

Tabbouleh Salad Recipe

Prep Time: 25 Minutes
Style: American
Cook Time: 0 Minutes
Difficulty: Difficult

2.8g
Protein

9.3g
Fat

3.9g
Fiber

149.5cal
Calories

INGREDIENTS

1/2 cup, dry, yield Bulgur

1 cup Tap Water

2 plum tomatoes Red Tomatoes

1 cucumber (8-1/4") Cucumber (with Peel)

3/4 cup Parsley

8 tablespoons Peppermint (Mint)

3 large Scallions or Spring Onions

1/4 cup Extra Virgin Olive Oil

1/4 cup Fresh Lemon Juice

1 teaspoon Salt

1/2 teaspoon Black Pepper

DIRECTIONS

1. Combine bulgur and water in a large heatproof dish; cover securely with plastic wrap and let stand until water is absorbed, approximately 15 minutes.

2. Line a sieve with cheesecloth or a dish towel, lay bulgur in it, and press hard using your hands to remove any extra water.

3. Add tomatoes, cucumber, parsley, mint, lemon juice, oil, scallions, salt, and pepper; mix gently to incorporate. Serve chilled or at room temperature.

Mediterranean Vegetable and Egg Salad Recipe

Prep Time: 15 Minutes
Style: Mediterranean/Greek
Cook Time: 0 Minutes
Difficulty: Moderate

10.7g
Protein

31.7g
Fat

2.5g
Fiber

371.7cal
Calories

INGREDIENTS

2 tablespoons Red Wine Vinegar

1 teaspoon Dijon Mustard

1/4 teaspoon Salt

1/4 teaspoon Black Pepper

1/3 cup Extra Virgin Olive Oil

1 14.5 oz jar Marinated Artichoke Hearts

1 cup Cherry Tomato

4 ounces Black Olives

1 tablespoon drained Capers

1 oz, raw, yield Red Onions

2 tablespoons Parsley

6 large Boiled Eggs

4 cups fresh romaine lettuce

DIRECTIONS
1. For the dressing: Combine vinegar, mustard, salt and pepper in a jar with a tight-fitting cover; shake once, add oil and shake violently to blend.
2. For the salad: Combine artichoke hearts, quartered tomatoes, sliced olives, capers, chopped onion and parsley in a large bowl; add 2 tablespoons of the dressing and toss to cover.
3. Place lettuce in a serving dish, top with artichoke mixture and sliced or chopped eggs, sprinkle with remaining dressing and serve.

Keto Caprese Salad Recipe

Prep Time: 10 Minutes
Style: Italian
Cook Time: 0 Minutes
Difficulty: Moderate

12.8g
Protein

22.7g
Fat

1.1g
Fiber

256.3cal
Calories

INGREDIENTS

5 Cherry Tomatoes

2 ounces Fresh Mozzarella

1 tablespoon Extra Virgin Olive Oil

1/4 tablespoon Balsamic Vinegar

1 tablespoon Basil, fresh, chopped

1/16 teaspoon Black Pepper, ground

1/16 teaspoon Salt

DIRECTIONS
1. Slice tomatoes and mozzarella.
2. Drizzle with olive oil and vinegar.
3. Julienne or cut the fresh basil leaves and put on top. Season with a touch of salt and pepper and serve immediately.

Italian Chopped Salad Recipe
Prep Time: 20 Minutes

Style: Italian

Cook Time: 0 Minutes

Difficulty: Difficult

29.6g

Protein

28.4g

Fat

4.6g

Fiber

420.4cal

Calories

INGREDIENTS

2 tablespoons Red Wine Vinegar

1 tablespoon Basil, fresh, chopped

1 tablespoon Parmesan Cheese, grated

1 teaspoon Dijon Mustard

1 tablespoon Olive Oil

1/2 cup Snap Peas, in pod, fresh, chopped

1 cup Cucumber, raw, sliced

10 each Cherry or Grape Tomato

2 ounces Mozzarella Cheese, fresh balls

1/2 package (4 oz) Hard Salami

4 ounces Chicken Roasted, dark and light meat

4 cups Romaine, raw, shredded

1 cup Baby Spinach

DIRECTIONS

1. Whisk together the vinegar, chopped basil, and Parmesan with the mustard. Slowly add the oil while whisking into a vinaigrette. Set aside.

2. Prepare veggies by slicing the peas, cucumber, tomatoes, mozzarella cheese, salami and cooked chicken into bite sized pieces.

3. Toss together the Romaine and spinach with the dressing. Top with the chopped veggies, meats and cheese. Serve immediately.

Grilled Chicken over Baby Spinach, Tomato and Avocado Salad Recipe
Prep Time: 5 Minutes

Style: American

Cook Time: 10 Minutes

Difficulty: Moderate

57g

Protein

35.2g

Fat

10.8g

Fiber

607.2cal

Calories

INGREDIENTS

1 serving Keto Sweet Mustard Dressing

6 ounces Chicken Breast Filet, skinless

2 cups Baby Spinach

1/2 large whole (3" diameter) Red Tomatoes

1/2 fruit without skin and seed California Avocados

DIRECTIONS

1. Preheat a grill and season chicken with salt and freshly ground black pepper.

2. Grill over medium heat until juices run clear and it is no longer pink in the middle.

3. Combine the baby spinach, tomato and avocado with the dressing. Top with cooked chicken and serve immediately.

Chapter 10: Vegan Recipe

83. Mushroom and Cauliflower Vegan Shepherds Pie

84. Vegan Cauliflower Pizza with Basil Pesto

85. Vegan Burrito Bowl

86. Vegan Mushroom Soup

87. Low-Carb Vegan Chow Mein

88. Creamy Tuscan Spaghetti Squash (Paleo, Vegan)

89. Sesame Ginger Tofu and Veggie Stir Fry

90.No Bean Chilli Recipe (Vegan)

91. Golden Baked Jicama Fries

Mushroom and Cauliflower Vegan Shepherds Pie

Prep Time: 30 minutes
Cook Time: 30 Minutes
Total Time: 1 hour

23g
Protein

11g
Fat

1212mg
Fiber

400 cal
Calories

INGREDIENTS

650 g cauliflower (1 ½ pounds)

2 tbsp olive oil

1 onion diced

2 medium sized carrots peeled and diced

1 celery stalk diced

3 cloves garlic chopped

10 g dried wild mushrooms reconstituted in 2 ½ tbsp boiling water (⅓ oz)

500 g mushrooms diced (1 pound)

1 tbsp thyme leaves roughly chopped

1 tbsp tomato paste

¼ cup red wine

1 cup vegetable stock

salt and pepper to taste

2 tbsp olive oil

3 tbsp nutritional yeast

1 tbsp dijon mustard

1 tsp salt

2 tsp thyme leaves

1 pinch ground nutmeg

DIRECTIONS

1. Preheat the oven to 200 celsius (400 fahrenheit).

2. Chop the cauliflower into about equal sized pieces and add to a big pot. Cover with water and bring to a boil. Season with salt and boil the cauliflower until soft. Drain.

3. Place a large frying pan over a medium heat. Add the olive oil, onion, carrots and celery. Cook until slightly brown and caramelized. Add the mushrooms in 6 sections, ensuring each batch is cooked before adding the next.

4. Remove the wild mushrooms from the boiling water, retaining the water, and coarsely chop. Add to the mushrooms along with the tomato paste. Increase the heat to medium-high and add the red wine. Cook until the red wine has nearly gone before adding the mushroom soaking liquid and vegetable stock. Reduce the heat to low and simmer for 5 to 10 minutes or until about half of the liquid has been absorbed. Remove from the heat.

5. Place the cauliflower in a food processor or high speed blender along with 2 tbsp olive oil, the nutritional yeast, mustard, salt and thyme leaves. Blend till smooth and taste. Adjust spices as desired and add the nutmeg and mix for a further minute.

6. Divide the mushrooms amongst 4 large ramekins and top with the cauliflower mash. Bake for 20 minutes or until gently browned.

Vegan Cauliflower Pizza with Basil Pesto
Prep Time: 20 minutes
Cook Time:1 hour 10 minutes
Total Time:1hour 30minutes
Servings: 4

7.7g
Protein

20g
Fat

5.5g
Fiber

245 cal
Calories

INGREDIENTS

For the cauliflower pizza base:

4 cups of cauliflower rice

2 tablespoon flaxseed meal

5 tablespoon water

1/3 cup almond flour

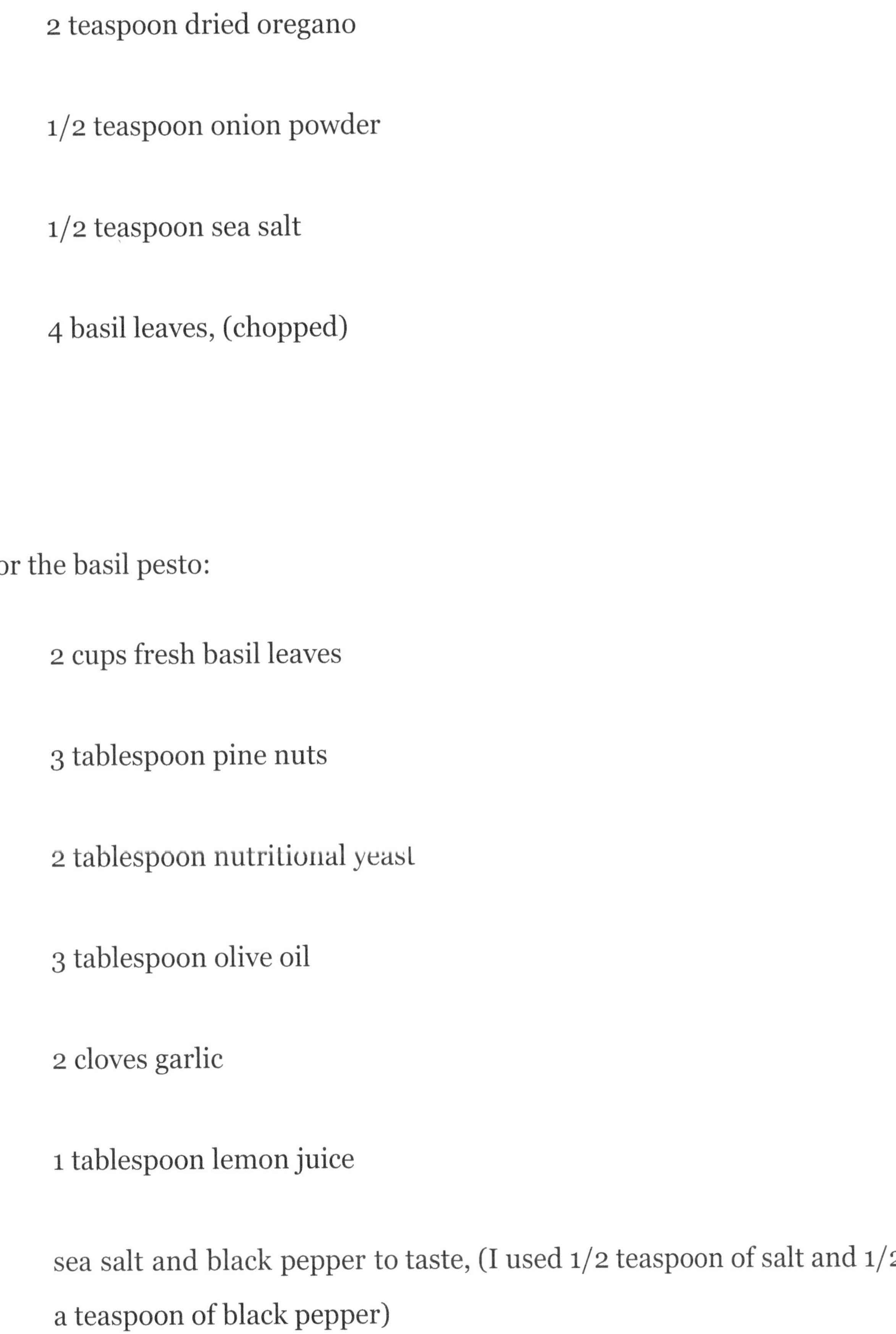

2 teaspoon dried oregano

1/2 teaspoon onion powder

1/2 teaspoon sea salt

4 basil leaves, (chopped)

For the basil pesto:

2 cups fresh basil leaves

3 tablespoon pine nuts

2 tablespoon nutritional yeast

3 tablespoon olive oil

2 cloves garlic

1 tablespoon lemon juice

sea salt and black pepper to taste, (I used 1/2 teaspoon of salt and 1/2 a teaspoon of black pepper)

DIRECTIONS

1. Preheat your oven to 375 F (190°C).

2. To prepare cauliflower rice from home, chop a big head of cauliflower into small florets. Grate these florets using a box grater with medium-sized holes or use a grater attachment on your food processor. Alternatively, you may purchase pre-riced cauliflower.

3. Bring a big saucepan of water to a boil and add the riced cauliflower. Mix and simmer for 5 minutes until the rice is mushy.

4. Drain the cauliflower rice using a fine mesh strainer or a dish towel. Once most of the water has drained, lay the rice aside to cool for 5 minutes.

5. While the cauliflower rice is cooling, combine the flaxseed meal and water and shape it into a ball. Set aside.

6. Wrap the cooled cauliflower rice in the dish towel and ring out as much water as you can. You want to eliminate as much moisture as possible.

7. Add the cauliflower rice, prepared flaxseed ball, almond flour, oregano, onion powder, sea salt, and chopped basil leaves to a large mixing bowl.

8. Use your hands to mix the items completely.

9. Spread the dough on a baking sheet sprinkled with gluten-free flour and shape into a circle. It should be around 1/2 inch (1.5 cm) thick with somewhat thicker edges.

10. Bake the crust for 30 minutes, then remove from the oven.

11. Add a thin layer of tomato sauce and your selected toppings. Bake for another 10-15 minutes until the sides are golden brown and the base is cooked through.

12. While the pizza is in the oven, combine all of the ingredients for the basil pesto into a food processor and pulse until they come together. If it isn't combining smoothly, add additional water.

13. Remove the pizza from the oven, pour some of the newly produced basil pesto over the pie, and serve hot.

Vegan Burrito Bowl
Prep Time: 10 minutes
Cook Time:30 minutes
Total Time:40 minutes

10g
Protein

16g
Fat

14g
Fiber

368 cal
Calories

INGREDIENTS
For the Roasted Sweet Potatoes
3 cups cubed sweet potato
1 tbsp olive oil
2 tsp smoked paprika
For the Veggie Bowls

1 tbsp avocado oil OR olive oil
1 large onion diced
2 cloves garlic minced
1 red bell pepper diced
2 tbsp tomato paste
1 tsp cumin
1 tsp garam masala
2 cups mushrooms sliced
3/4 cup corn (optional - leave out for paleo / Whole30 / low carb / keto)
2 tbsp coconut aminos
1/2 cup canned black beans drained and rinsed (optional - leave out for paleo / Whole30 / low carb / keto)
Juice of 1 lime
For Serving
1 cup cauliflower rice
2 cups lettuce chopped
1 cup tomatoes diced
1 cup cucumber diced
1 large avocado mashed
Extra lime juice to garnish

DIRECTIONS

1. Preheat the oven to 400°F. Line a large baking sheet with parchment paper. Spread out the sweet potatoes and sprinkle with oil, salt and smoked paprika and roast in a preheated oven for 20-25 minutes, until crispy, turning halfway through.

2. Meanwhile, heat olive oil in a big skillet/pan over a medium-high heat.

3. Add the onion, garlic, bell peppers, tomato paste, cumin and garam masala. Cook for 5 minutes, until the veggies soften.

4. Next, add the mushrooms and corn (if using), simmering for 3-4 minutes longer.

5. Add the coconut aminos and black beans, if using. Squeeze in the lime juice and simmer for 5 minutes, stirring regularly, until the beans soften.
6. Cook the cauliflower rice till cooked and create the guacamole. Mash avocado with the remainder of the lime juice and little salt and pepper.

7. Serve the sweet potato and black beans in a dish combined with the cauliflower rice, lettuce, tomatoes, cucumber, avocado and additional lime juice.

Vegan Mushroom Soup

Prep Time: 10 Minutes

Style: American

Cook Time: 45 Minutes

6g
Protein

16g
Fat

2g
Fiber

206 cal
Calories

EQUIPMENTS

6-Quart Dutch Oven

Blender

INGREDIENTS

3-4 tbsp low-sodium vegetable broth (for sauteing)

1 medium yellow onion sliced

5 garlic cloves minced

¾ tsp dried thyme

½ tsp himalayan pink sea salt

¼ tsp black pepper

1.5 lbs cremini mushrooms sliced

8 oz shiitake mushrooms (fresh or frozen)

4 cups low-sodium vegetable broth
(1) 14 oz can coconut milk (discard the water, try to only use the creamy part)

2 tbsp chives sliced

DIRECTIONS

1. In a 6-quart dutch oven over medium heat, sauté the chopped onions in 3-4 tbsp vegetable broth until transparent, approximately 10 minutes. Add 5 cloves of minced garlic, ¾ tsp dried thyme, ½ tsp salt, and ¼ tsp black pepper. Give it a toss and let it simmer for 2 more minutes.

2. Add the cut cremini mushrooms and frozen shiitake mushrooms. Let the mushrooms cook for 15 minutes or until they're tender.

3. Transfer the mushroom mixture to a big blender cup and add 2-3 cups (depending on how large the blender cup is) of vegetable broth. Blend on high until the mixture is smooth and creamy.

4. Pour the combined mushroom puree back into the dutch oven and whisk in the remaining vegetable broth. Next, add the canned coconut milk, but try to just pour in the creamy white portion and discard (or preserve for a smoothie) the watery liquid.

5. Stir the soup to incorporate the coconut milk with the mushroom purée until it's totally combined. Let the soup stew for 5-10 more minutes over medium heat until it's hot and beginning to bubble.

6. Serve and garnish each dish with fresh chives.

Low-Carb Vegan Chow Mein

Prep Time: 15 Minutes

Style: Asian

Cook Time: 15 Minutes

18g
Protein

7g
Fat

4g
Fiber

197 cal
Calories

INGREDIENTS

6 medium zucchinis, approx. 1500 g 1 tsp sesame oil

4 carrots, peeled and chopped into thin diagonal slices

4 cloves garlic, minced

6 stalks of green onion, chopped

2–3 cups cabbage, thinly sliced (napa, savoy or sui choy)

1 tsp coriander

1 tsp ginger

3 tbsp soy sauce (use tamari or coconut aminos for gluten-free)

3 tbsp hoisin sauce (use gluten-free such as Joyce Chen, if needed)

2 tbsp roasted red chili paste

3 tbsp vegetable broth

DIRECTIONS

1. Spiralize the zucchini, put in a strainer, sprinkle with salt and leave aside. Let it alone for 10 minutes then lay all the zoodles in a dish towel, wrap up the ends and thoroughly press out all the extra water. Do not miss this step!

2. Make the sauce by whisking together the soy sauce, hoisin sauce, red chili paste and vegetable broth. Set aside.

3. Heat the sesame oil in a large, non-stick pan over medium high heat.

4. Add the carrots and garlic and sauté for 5-10 minutes, stirring.

5. Add the green onion and cabbage and continue cooking until the cabbage has wilted.

6. Stir in the coriander and ginger.

7. Add the zucchini noodles and sauté for roughly 5 minutes.

8. Stir in the sauce.

9. Serve.

Creamy Tuscan Spaghetti Squash (Paleo, Vegan)

Prep Time: 10 Minutes

Style: American

Cook Time: 1 hour

4g
Protein

10g
Fat

4g
Fiber

171 cal
Calories

INGREDIENTS

1 medium spaghetti squash, roasted, about 3 cups

3/4 cup full-fat canned coconut milk

2 cloves garlic, minced

2 cups baby spinach

1/3 cup sun-dried tomatoes, drained

1/2 cup artichoke hearts

1 tsp dried parsley

1/2 tsp sea salt, to taste

1/4 tsp black pepper

DIRECTIONS

1. Begin by roasting the spaghetti squash by following my instructions on How To Roast Spaghetti Squash or Instant Pot Spaghetti Squash.
2. Once the spaghetti squash has completed roasting and is cool enough to handle, use a fork to loosen the spaghetti strands and set them in a big bowl (or large 4-cup measuring cup if you have one).
3. Heat the coconut milk in a medium-sized pan over medium-high heat until it comes to a full boil.
4. Add the garlic and sauté, stirring regularly until garlic is extremely fragrant, approximately 3 minutes.
5. Add the spaghetti squash to the saucepan and stir thoroughly. Add the baby spinach and cover. Cook until spinach has wilted.
6. Remove the cover and toss in the sun-dried tomatoes, artichoke hearts, dried parsley, sea salt and black pepper. Continue cooking

another 2 to 3 minutes until all ingredients are well-combined and the sauce is lovely and thick.

7. Serve with your favorite entrée, and enjoy! You may also add your preferred protein such as chicken breasts, rotisserie chicken, shrimp, or ground turkey to the dish.

Sesame Ginger Tofu and Veggie Stir Fry

Prep Time: 25 Minutes

Cook Time: 15 minutes

13g
Protein

12g
Fat

3.2g
Fiber

233 cal
Calories

INGREDIENTS

STIR FRY:

1 (14 ounce) package extra firm tofu

1 tablespoon cornstarch

½ teaspoon kosher salt

3 tablespoons high heat oil (such as avocado)

2 ½ cups green beans, cut into 1-inch pieces

1 cup baby carrots, cut lengthwise

SAUCE:

1 tablespoons sesame oil

1 ½ tablespoon grated ginger

1 ½ tablespoons minced garlic

1 tablespoons rice vinegar

3 tablespoons soy sauce (or GF tamari)

¼ teaspoon red pepper flakes

3 tablespoons brown sugar

1 tablespoon cornstarch

2 tablespoons water

DIRECTIONS

TOFU: Drain tofu from packing. Place tofu on a platter with a folded tea towel. Place another tea towel on top (in the form of the tofu) followed by another plate and a hefty cast iron pan or metal cans. Or just use a tofu press. Let tofu dry for 15-20 minutes or up to 1 hour. Then, cut into ¾-1 inch cubes and throw in 1 tablespoon of cornstarch and ½ teaspoon of salt in a zip-top bag until coated.

BLEND: While the tofu is drying, make the sauce. Combine sauce ingredients in a blender until totally smooth (see notes) Set aside.

CRISPY TOFU: In a wok or large nonstick pan over medium-high heat, add 2 teaspoons of oil. Add tofu and let cook for 3-7 minutes. Flip tofu as required to brown on both sides. Add 2 tablespoons of prepared sauce and let to heat until the sauce covers the tofu;

approximately 2-3 minutes. When the tofu is caramelized, transfer to a dish.

STIR FRY:Add the remaining tablespoon of oil to the pan, if required. Toss in vegetables and cook for 3-4 minutes, stirring as required to desired doneness. Add tofu back to the skillet. Stir the sauce to blend and pour it in. Stir to coat. Cook for a further 1-2 minutes or until the tofu soaks up the sauce.

SERVE: Serve warm with rice, quinoa, noodles, cauliflower rice, or on its own. The tofu will lose its firmness as it sits. Best when eaten fresh.

No Bean Chilli Recipe (Vegan)

Prep Time:10 Minutes

Cook Time: 31 minutes

13g
Protein

28g
Fat

8g
Fiber

353 cal
Calories

INGREDIENTS

2 tbsp extra virgin olive Oil

5 stalks celery finely diced

2 cloves garlic minced

1 1/2 tsp ground cinnamon

2 tsp chili powder

4 tsp ground cumin

1 ½ tsp smoked paprika

2 peppers large chipotle in adobo minced

2 green bell peppers finely diced

2 zucchini diced

8 oz cremini mushrooms minced in a food processor

1 1/2 tbsp tomato paste

1 15 oz can diced tomatoes

3 cups water

1/2 cup coconut milk

2 1/2 cups soy meat crumbled

1 cup raw walnuts minced

1 tbsp unsweetened cocoa powder

Salt and pepper to taste

TO SERVE:

2 tbsp Fresh cilantro leaves

1 Avocado sliced

2 tbsp Sliced radishes

DIRECTIONS

1. Heat the oil in a big saucepan over medium heat. Add the celery and simmer for 4 minutes. Add in the garlic, cinnamon, chili powder, cumin and paprika and stir until fragrant, for another 2 minutes.
2. Add the bell peppers, zucchini, mushrooms and simmer for 5 minutes.
3. Add the chipotle, tomato paste, tomatoes, water, coconut milk, soy meat, walnuts and cocoa powder. Reduce the heat to medium-low and simmer for approximately 20-25 minutes until thick and the veggies are tender.
4. Season with salt and pepper, to taste. Top with avocado, radishes, and cilantro.

Golden Baked Jicama Fries

Prep Time: 20 Minutes

Style: American

Cook Time: 50 minutes

5g
Protein

58g
Carb

32g
Fiber

250 cal
Calories

INGREDIENTS

2 1/2 cups (20 fluid ounces) water

1 1/2 teaspoons salt, divided

15 ounces jicama *(whole or pre-packaged)*

1 Tablespoon + 2 teaspoons (25 milliliters) avocado oil *or* olive oil

1/2 teaspoon ground turmeric

1/4 teaspoon garlic powder

1/4 teaspoon paprika

1/8 teaspoon onion powder

2 teaspoons fresh parsley, finely chopped

DIRECTIONS

Prepare: Preheat the oven to 400 degrees F and line the baking sheet with parchment paper. If using a full jicama, using a vegetable peeler, remove skin off the jicama. Slice peeled jicama into fries. (You may omit this step if using pre-peeled and pre-sliced jicama.)

Boil Jicama: To a medium-sized saucepan over high heat, add water and ½ teaspoon salt and bring to a boil. Add sliced jicama, cover saucepan, and simmer for 15 minutes. Remove the saucepan from heat and then drain the water.

Season Boiled Jicama: Transfer jicama to a large mixing bowl, sprinkle with oil and add remaining 1 teaspoon salt and the spices. Toss using a spoon or tongs until the jicama is well covered in oil and spices.

Bake: Transfer seasoned jicama onto the prepared baking sheet in a single layer. Bake for 40 minutes, turning over each fry after approximately 20 minutes.

Serve: Remove from the oven and let cool slightly before garnishing with chopped fresh parsley.

Air Fryer Instructions: Cook in a preheated air fryer at 400 degrees F. Be sure you follow the directions to boil them first. Then, air fry them in batches, and be cautious not to overcrowd them in the air fryer basket.

Meal Prepping Instructions: To meal prep these, peel and slice the jicama and then boil it. After this, transfer the fries to a paper towel-lined plate to drain most of the excess water and moisture, and then transfer the boiled fries to an airtight storage container. When you're ready to properly prepare them, proceed with the remaining preparation procedures (seasoning and baking).

Refrigerator Storage: Store the made fries in an airtight container in the refrigerator for 3-4 days.

Chapter 11: Vegetarian Recipe

92. Aubergine & chickpea stew

93. Roasted aubergine & tomato curry

94. Bean & halloumi stew

95. Coconut & squash dhansak

96. Spiced lentil & butternut squash soup

97. Sweet potato & peanut curry

98. Herb omelet with fried tomatoes

99. Aubergine, tomato & Parmesan bake (Melanzane alla Parmigiana)

100. West Indian spiced aubergine curry

101. Vegetarian Thai green curry

Aubergine & chickpea stew
Prep Time: 15 Minutes
Cook Time: 8-10 hours (plus overnight soaking)

Difficulty: Moderate

11g
Protein

10g
Fat

12g
Fiber

266 cal
Calories

INGREDIENTS

- 200g dried chickpeas, soaked for 6-8 hours

- 2 tbsp extra virgin olive oil, plus extra to serve (optional)

- 2 onions, finely sliced

- 6 garlic cloves, crushed

- 1 tbsp baharat

- 1 tsp ground cinnamon

- 1 small bunch of flat-leaf parsley, stalks finely chopped, leaves roughly chopped, to serve

3 medium aubergines, sliced into 2cm rounds

2 x 400g cans chopped tomatoes

1 lemon, juiced

50g pine nuts, toasted, to serve

pitta breads or flatbreads, to serve (optional)

DIRECTIONS

1. Drain the chickpeas and bring to the boil in a pan of salted water. Cook for 10 minutes, then drain.

2. Heat the oil in a frying pan over a medium heat and cook the onions for 10 minutes, or until starting to soften. Stir in the garlic, baharat and cinnamon and simmer for 1 min. Tip the onion mixture into a slow cooker and add the chickpeas, parsley stems, aubergines, tomatoes and a can of water. Season. Cover and simmer on high for 2 hrs, then switch the heat to low and cook for 6-8 hours longer until the mixture has reduced somewhat and the chickpeas and aubergines are wonderfully soft.

3. Stir in the lemon juice, then distribute over the pine nuts and parsley leaves. Drizzle over some more olive oil and serve with pitta breads or flatbreads, if you want.

Roasted aubergine & tomato curry

Prep Time: 15 Minutes

Cook Time: 45 minutes

Difficulty: Moderate

5g
Protein

26g
Fat

7g
Fiber

331 cal
Calories

INGREDIENTS

600g aubergine, or baby aubergines sliced into rounds

3 tbsp olive oil

2 onions, finely sliced

2 garlic cloves, crushed

1 tsp garam masala

1 tsp turmeric

1 tsp ground coriander

400ml can chopped tomatoes

400ml can coconut milk

pinch of sugar (optional)

½ small pack coriander, roughly chopped

rice or chapatis, to serve

DIRECTIONS

1. Heat oven to 200C/180C fan/gas 6. Toss the aubergines in a roasting tray with 2 tbsp olive oil, season generously and spread out. Roast for 20 minutes or till dark golden and supple.

2. Heat the remaining oil in an ovenproof skillet or flameproof casserole dish and sauté the onions over a medium heat for 5-6 minutes until softened. Stir in the garlic and spices, for a few moments till the spices unleash their fragrances.

3. Tip in the tomatoes, coconut milk and roasted aubergines, and bring to a slow boil. Simmer for 20-25 minutes, lifting the top for the last 5 mins to thicken the sauce. Add a little salt if you prefer, and a touch of sugar if it needs it. Stir through most of the coriander. Serve over rice or with chapatis, sprinkling with the leftover coriander.

Bean & halloumi stew

Prep Time: 5 Minutes

Cook Time: 20 minutes

Difficulty: Moderate

19g
Protein

25g
Fat

14g
Fiber

468 cal
Calories

INGREDIENTS

3 tbsp olive oil

1 onion, thinly sliced

1 red pepper, thinly sliced

2 garlic cloves, crushed

3 tbsp red chili pesto, sundried tomato pesto or vegan alternative

1 heaped tsp ground coriander

400g can mixed beans, drained and rinsed

400g can chopped tomatoes

½ x 250g block halloumi, sliced

½ small bunch of coriander, finely chopped

garlic bread, to serve (optional)

DIRECTIONS

1. Heat 2 tbsp of oil in a frying pan over a medium heat. Add the onion and pepper, along with a sprinkle of salt and cook for 10 minutes or until softened. Add the garlic, pesto and ground coriander, and simmer for 1 min. Tip in the beans and tomatoes together with ½ can of water, then bring to a boil and cook uncovered for 10 minutes.

2. Add the remaining oil to a separate frying pan over a medium heat. Fry the halloumi for 2 minutes on each side or until golden brown.

3. Taste the beans for flavor, then pour into deep bowls. Top with the halloumi and distribute over the chopped coriander. Serve with garlic bread, if you prefer.

Coconut & squash dhansak

Prep Time: 5 Minutes

Cook Time: 15 minutes

Difficulty: Moderate

9g
Protein

17g
Fat

7g
Fiber

320 cal
Calories

INGREDIENTS

1 tbsp vegetable oil

500g butternut squash (about 1 small squash), peeled and chopped into bite-sized chunks (or buy a pack of ready-prepared to save time), see tip, below left

100g frozen chopped onions

4 heaped tbsp mild curry paste (we used korma)

400g can chopped tomatoes

400g can light coconut milk

mini naan bread, to serve

400g can lentils, drained

200g bag baby spinach

150ml coconut yogurt (we used Rachel's Organic), plus extra to serve

DIRECTIONS

1. Heat the oil in a big pan. Put the squash in a basin with a splash of water. Cover with cling film and microwave on High for 10 minutes or until soft. Meanwhile, add the onions to the heated oil and sauté for a few minutes until tender. Add the curry paste, tomatoes and coconut milk, and cook for 10 minutes until thickened to a rich sauce.

2. Warm the naan bread in a low oven or in the toaster. Drain any liquid from the squash, then add to the sauce with the lentils, spinach and some spices. Simmer for a further 2-3 minutes to wilt the spinach, then whisk in the coconut yogurt. Serve with the heated naan and a dollop of additional yogurt.

Spiced lentil & butternut squash soup
Prep Time: 10 Minutes
Cook Time: 40 minutes
Difficulty: Moderate

6g
Protein

5g
Fat

3g
Fiber

167 cal
Calories

INGREDIENTS

2 tbsp olive oil

2 onions, finely chopped

2 garlic cloves, crushed

¼ tsp hot chili powder

1 tbsp ras el hanout

1 butternut squash, peeled and cut into 2cm pieces

100g red lentils

1l hot vegetable stock

1 small bunch coriander, leaves chopped, plus extra to serve

dukkah (see tip) and natural yogurt, to serve

DIRECTIONS

1. Heat the oil in a large flameproof casserole dish or saucepan over a medium-high heat. Fry the onions with a bit of salt for 7 minutes, or until softened and barely caramelized. Add the garlic, chili and ras el hanout, and simmer for 1 min longer.

2. Stir in the squash and lentils. Pour over the stock and season to taste. Bring to the boil, then lower the heat to a simmer and cook, covered, for 25 minutes or until the squash is tender. Blitz the soup with a stick blender until smooth, then season to taste. freeze, allow it to cool fully and transfer to big freezer proof bags.

3. Stir in the coriander leaves and spoon the soup into dishes. Serve topped with the dukkah, yogurt and additional coriander leaves.

Sweet potato & peanut curry
Prep Time: 15 Minutes
Cook Time: 45 minutes
Difficulty: Moderate

6g
Protein

25g
Fat

7g
Fiber

387 cal
Calories

INGREDIENTS

1 tbsp coconut oil

1 onion, chopped

2 garlic cloves, grated

thumb-sized piece ginger, grated

3 tbsp Thai red curry paste (check the label to make sure it's vegetarian/ vegan)

1 tbsp smooth peanut butter

500g sweet potato, peeled and cut into chunks

400ml can coconut milk

200g bag spinach

1 lime, juiced

cooked rice, to serve (optional)

dry roasted peanuts, to serve (optional)

DIRECTIONS

1. Melt 1 tbsp coconut oil in a saucepan over a medium heat and soften 1 chopped onion for 5 minutes. Add 2 grated garlic cloves and a grated thumb-sized piece of ginger, and simmer for 1 min until aromatic.

2. Stir in 3 tbsp Thai red curry paste, 1 tbsp smooth peanut butter and 500g sweet potato, peeled and sliced into bits, then add 400ml coconut milk and 200ml water.

3. Bring to the boil, turn down the heat and simmer, uncovered, for 25-30 minutes or until the sweet potato is tender.

4. Stir over 200g spinach and the juice of 1 lime, and season thoroughly. Serve over cooked rice, and if you want some crunch, sprinkle over a few dry toasted peanuts.

Herb omelet with fried tomatoes
Prep Time: 5 mins
Cook Time:5 mins

Difficulty: Moderate

17g
Protein

1g
Fat

1g
Fiber

204 cal
Calories

INGREDIENTS

  1 tsp olive oil

  3 tomatoes, halved

  4 large eggs

  1 tbsp chopped parsley

  1 tbsp chopped basil

DIRECTIONS

1. Heat the oil in a small non-stick frying pan, then sauté the tomatoes cut-side down until beginning to soften and color. Meanwhile, whisk the eggs with the herbs and lots of freshly ground black pepper in a small dish.

2. Scoop the tomatoes from the skillet and place them on two serving dishes. Pour the egg mixture into the pan and swirl gently with a wooden spoon so the egg that sets on the base of the pan slides to let the uncooked egg to flow into the area. Stop stirring when it's almost done to enable it to set into an omelet. Cut into four and serve with the tomatoes.

Aubergine, tomato & Parmesan bake (Melanzane alla Parmigiana)

Prep Time: 10 mins
Cook Time:50 mins
Difficulty: Moderate

10g
Protein

17g
Fat

5g

Fiber

225 cal

Calories

INGREDIENTS

2 garlic cloves, crushed

6 tbsp olive oil

2 x 400g cans chopped tomatoes

2 tbsp tomato purée

4 aubergines, cut into long, 5mm thick slices

85g parmesan (or vegetarian alternative), freshly grated

20g pack basil, leaves torn

1 egg, beaten

DIRECTIONS

1. Heat oven to 200C/fan 180C/gas 6. In a small pan, stir together the garlic and 4 tbsp of the olive oil. Cook over a high heat for 3 minutes, tip in the tomatoes, then simmer for 8 mins, stirring every now and again. Stir in the tomato purée.

2. Meanwhile, heat a griddle pan until extremely hot. Brush a couple of the aubergines with a little oil, then add to the pan. Cook over a high fire until fully browned and cooked through, approximately 5-7 minutes. Turn them halfway through cooking. Lift onto kitchen paper and do the next batch.

3. When all the aubergines are cooked, arrange a couple of them in the bottom of an ovenproof dish, then spread over some sauce. Sprinkle with Parmesan and basil leaves. Add seasoning, then continue this procedure with the remaining ingredients. Finally, pour the egg over the top, sprinkle over a little more Parmesan, then bake for 20 minutes or until the topping is brown.

West Indian spiced aubergine curry
Prep Time: 30 mins
Cook Time: 15 mins
Difficulty: Moderate

4g
Protein

9g
Fat

7g

Fiber

157 cal

Calories

INGREDIENTS

1 tsp ground cumin

1 tsp ground coriander

½ tsp ground turmeric

1 large aubergine

2 tbsp tomato purée

½ green chili, finely chopped

1 cm piece ginger, peeled and finely chopped

2 tsp caster sugar

½-1 tbsp rapeseed oil

3 spring onions, chopped

½ bunch of coriander, shredded

cooked rice, natural yogurt or vegan alternative, roti and lime wedges, to serve

DIRECTIONS

1. Mix the dry spices and 1 tsp salt together in a basin and keep aside.

2. Slice the aubergine into 1cm rounds, then slice both sides of each round with the point of a sharp knife. Rub with the spice mix until fully covered (you should use all of the mix), then move to a board. Put 150ml water in the empty spice bowl with the tomato purée, chili, ginger and sugar. Set aside.

3. Heat the oil in a large non-stick frying pan over a medium heat and put the aubergine in the pan, overlapping the rounds if desired. Fry for 5 minutes on each side, or until golden. Add the liquid mix from the bowl, bring to a simmer, cover and cook for 15-20 minutes, turning the aubergine periodically until it's cooked through. If it feels dry, you may need to add up to 100 ml extra water to make it saucier. Season.

4. Scatter over the spring onions and coriander, and serve with rice, yogurt, roti and lime wedges for squeezing over.

Vegetarian Thai green curry
Prep Time: 15 mins
Cook Time: 40 mins
Difficulty: Moderate

6g
Protein

26g
Fat

7g
Fiber

339 cal
Calories

INGREDIENTS

2 tbsp vegetable oil

3 shallots, finely sliced

4 tbsp Thai green curry paste

1 red chili, deseeded and finely chopped

350g butternut squash, peeled and cut into 1.5cm cubes

1 large red pepper, deseeded and cut into thick slices

400g can full fat coconut milk

5 lime leaves

150g mangetout

100g baby corn. halved lengthways

1 small bunch coriander, roughly chopped

cooked rice and lime wedges, to serve

DIRECTIONS

1. Heat the oil in a big flameproof casserole dish with a tight-fitting cover. Add the shallots with a big teaspoon of salt and cook for 7-10 minutes over a medium heat until softened and starting to caramelize. Add the curry paste and chile to the dish and sauté for 2 minutes. Tip in the squash and pepper, then whisk into the coconut milk along with 200ml water. Add the lime leaves, cover and simmer for 15-20 minutes or until the squash is soft.

2. Stir the mangetout and baby corn through the curry, then re-cover, cooking over a medium-low heat for a further 5 minutes or until the veg is just cooked. Season and toss through half the coriander. Remove the lime leaves and discard. Spoon the curry into deep bowls, sprinkle with the remaining coriander and serve with rice and lime wedges for squeezing over.

Chapter 12: Conclusion

In conclusion, the Atkins Diet book for beginners offers a promising pathway to improved health, sustainable weight loss, and overall well being. With its emphasis on low-carbohydrate, high-fat eating, the Atkins Diet challenges conventional dietary wisdom and provides a compelling alternative for those seeking to transform their lives through nutrition.

Throughout this book, I've explored the principles and phases of the Atkins Diet, delving into its history, guidelines, and practical tips for success. I've provided a diverse array of delicious recipes tailored specifically for beginners, ensuring that anyone embarking on the Atkins journey has the tools and resources they need to thrive.

As you embark on your Atkins journey, remember that sustainable change takes time and patience. Listen to your body, stay committed to your goals, and don't be afraid to seek support when needed. Whether you're looking to shed a few pounds, improve your energy levels, or simply adopt a healthier way of eating, the Atkins Diet can help you achieve your aspirations and unlock your full potential.

With dedication, perseverance, and a commitment to prioritizing your health, you have the power to transform your life from the inside out. Embrace the journey, savor the experience, and revel in the joy of discovering a new way of nourishing your body, mind, and spirit.

Here's to your health, happiness, and success on the Atkins Diet and beyond. Bon appétit!

Reviews

Dear readers, if you've had the chance to dive into 'Atkins Diet Book for Beginners 2024' by Sébastien Quenneville, I'd love to hear your thoughts! Your reviews help me improve and inspire others to embark on their own journey to better health. Please take a moment to share your feedback and experiences with me.